# Managing In An

Edited By William F. Minogue, MD

# Academic Health Care

An ACPE Publication

# Environment

# Managing In An

Edited By William F. Minogue, MD

# Academic Health Care

# Environment

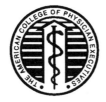

**American College of Physician Executives**
Two Urban Centre
Suite 200
4890 West Kennedy Boulevard
Tampa, Florida 33609
813/287-2000

ISBN: 0-924674-18-0

Library of Congress Card Number: 92-074401

Printed in the United States of America by Lithocolor, Tampa, Florida.

# Foreword

Although our great national academic health centers are a part of the nation's health care delivery system, they are also apart from it in many ways. Unlike most other provider organizations, academic institutions have multiple, often conflicting roles. They are providers of some of the most exquisitely complicated and technological health care services available at any given point in time. That unique role springs from the academic health center's responsibilities as a research organization, operating on the shifting forward boundaries of health care delivery. At the same time, these institutions are the source of training and education for tomorrow's health care providers, most notably physicians but also nurses, pharmacists, and a host of other health care professionals.

It is not an easy role to play, and there is no end to the list of critics. Those who receive services are, all at the same time, patients, "educational material," and research subjects. They may be pleased at the quality of the services they receive, but they are often critical of the manner in which the services are delivered. Like others in the health care system, our academic health centers must rely on funds for their operations from the full range of payers, and then add a new set of actors for the research and teaching elements. All these actors are critics as well as supporters.

Complicating the picture are existing and gathering forces that are inexorably changing the way that health is viewed and delivered in this country. Competition heads the list, and our academic health centers are not well-positioned for a competitive battle for patients. Yet patients, in the final analysis, are the most basic commodity for academic health centers, as they are for all the other elements in the system.

So how does one manage in this seeming morass? Can such a system be managed at all? In this new book from the College, William F. Minogue, MD, Chair of the College's Society on Academic Health Centers when the book was designed and written, has assembled an outstanding group of experts to delineate both what defines the academic health center and what will be required to manage these institutions successfully in this fast-changing world. No one who hopes to survive and prosper in the years ahead in managing the provision of academic medicine can afford to be without the knowledge that this book imparts. And the book confirms what we already know. The U.S. academic health system can and will be managed successfully.

*Roger Schenke*
*Executive Vice President*
*American College of Physician Executives*
*Tampa, Florida*
*September 1, 1992*

i

# Preface

Like Topsy, the academic health center (AHC) was not planned. "It just growed." AHCs have evolved to their present state since the Flexner report appeared early in this century. During World War I, entire faculties established field hospitals in Europe. In World War II, great advances were made in battlefield casualty management, and medical school faculty members were large contributors to the effort. The second half of this century has brought rapid advances in science and technology. As a nation, we have clearly evolved the finest medical education system in the world.

Yet, with all of the great advances to which academic health centers have been a party and with their enormous contribution to the public health, why are AHCs troubled today?

■ They are all competing for the same, limited research funds.

■ For more than two decades, they have been producing too many specialists and not enough primary physicians.

■ AHCs are expensive to operate.

■ Federal, state, and philanthropic support is dwindling.

■ They are frequently situated in urban centers and provide an enormous amount of uncompensated indigent care.

■ Faculty members, department chairs, and deans are promoted largely because of their research prowess.

■ The leadership of academic health centers is frequently lacking in management training and expertise (the American College of Physician Executives has a very small number of members from the academic community).

■ Faculty practice plans have become a "cash cow," placing a heavy demand on the faculty to generate income at the expense of teaching and research.

■ AHCs are frequently perceived by society as narcissistic and as serving the facility's interests first.

■ They are traditionally weak in strategic planning, particularly as it relates to community needs and to "customer" satisfaction.

There is, however, hope for the future.

■ The Association of American Medical Colleges' leadership has recently focused on the responsibility of AHCs to influence physician specialty mix and distribution.

■ Academic health centers have become proactive in the debate over health care reform.

Wilson and McLaughlin have provided this book with a marvelous chapter on strategic planning. If their views were adopted by the majority of AHCs, medical education would progress mightily toward improvement.

Deming, Nolan, and Batalden have enhanced our thinking about the organization as a system (see figure below). Frequently, AHCs have concentrated on the "production process," with far too little time and energy expended on the "aim" (i.e., why do we exist, what is the societal need for our products, what is our mission, who are our customers, and what are their needs?).

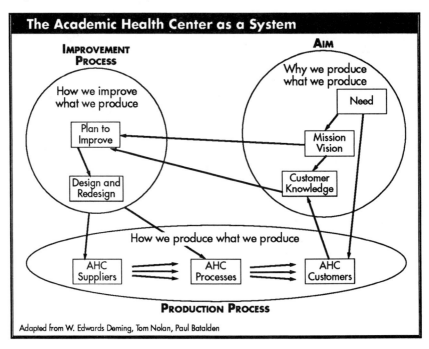

**The Academic Health Center as a System**

IMPROVEMENT PROCESS

How we improve what we produce

Plan to Improve

Design and Redesign

AIM

Why we produce what we produce

Need

Mission Vision

Customer Knowledge

How we produce what we produce

AHC Suppliers → AHC Processes → AHC Customers

PRODUCTION PROCESS

Adapted from W. Edwards Deming, Tom Nolan, Paul Batalden

The "improvement process' has also been problematic in academia. It has often been stated that changing a curriculum is, politically, about as easy as moving the town cemetery. As a senior physician with a son who is a recent medical school graduate, I am amazed at how little the process of educating a physician has changed over the past 30 years. Properly focused, AHCs, the National Board of Medical Examiners, the specialty societies, and the specialty boards can realign the medical education enterprise. They will have to integrate their activities on the basis of public health needs and a common vision for the future.

Enjoy this wonderful monograph. The authors have provided us with extremely valuable information and insights. AHCs are in the best leadership position to fundamentally change the quality of health care in the long run. We hope this monograph will serve as a reference guide as the nation struggles to reform the health care system.

***William F. Minogue, MD***
*Vice President for Clinical Affairs*
*Bon Secours Health System,. Inc.*
*Marriotsville, Md.*
*October 1, 1992*

# Table of Contents

# Table of Contents

# Chapter 1

# Academia and the Health Care System

*by Charles C. Lobeck, MD*

 The relationship of the system of professional education and research to the health and medical care of the people of the United States is complex and important. Management of this academic enterprise will be one of the keys to the success of the U.S. health care system. Formal management training of the leaders of this segment of the health care delivery system is not yet common but it will be one of the major ingredients for the system's success. To introduce the reader to this complex system, terms will be defined and the kinds of academic organizations that contribute to the health care delivery system will be discussed.

## Definitions

### Academia

The term academia, as used in higher education, connotes traditional colleges and universities. Health professional schools do not always exist in close relationship to these institutions. Some are alone or in consortia with other health professional schools, called medical or health universities. Even when part of traditional universities, health professional schools may be located away from the campuses of their parent universities and linked only through governance relationships. Therefore, the term academia as used in this chapter does not refer to higher education as a whole, but to health professional schools and the health care institutions, mainly hospitals, that provide the environment for professional education.

### Health Professional Schools

The dominant school in health professional education is the medical school. There were 126 fully accredited medical schools in the United States in 1991[1]; 73 were under public control and 53 were privately owned. With the exception of graduates of foreign medical schools, these schools are the origin of medical care providers in the United States. The development of medical education and the reasons for its dominance of health professional education in the United States have been the subject of several excellent scholarly reviews.[2,3] Nursing and other professional schools, other than dental schools, confer undergraduate degrees as their primary professional degrees. These schools often are not part of universities but are controlled by hospitals, technical schools, or undergraduate schools and colleges. These institutions and their contributions will not be considered here.

## Academic Health Center

The academic health center (AHC), an organization that has seen its greatest development since World War II, serves as the main direct link of academia with the health care delivery system. It is defined by the Association of Academic Health Centers as the consortium of a medical school, osteopathic or allopathic, with at least one other health professional school or program and one or more teaching hospitals. In 1991, there were 124 American and Canadian AHCs that met this definition; 104 were members of the Association. Consortia of hospitals with a medical school, but without other health professional schools, are often termed academic medical centers. Fewer and fewer of these exist as medical schools have developed relationships with other health professional schools. The term AHC will be used for both academic medical and health centers.

It is through AHCs that academia has its most focused relation to the health care delivery system. Medical schools without some relationship to hospitals do not exist. Hospitals, of course, may or may not be associated with medical schools and other professional schools.

## Teaching Hospitals

Teaching hospitals are those hospitals that, in addition to their mission of providing care to their communities, have responsibility for at least some clinical education for physicians in training. Some of them have graduate medical education (GME) as their only educational mission. GME is defined as training following the MD or DO degree leading to certification in a specialty of medicine. Trainees are called residents throughout their training period, which is a minimum of 3 years. In 1989, 17.5 percent (963 of 5,497) of short-term, nonfederal hospitals had these programs. In that same year, 19.1 percent (1,054 of 5,497) of U.S. hospitals,[4] not necessarily the same hospitals as those with GME, were affiliated with medical schools. In addition, 169 or 50 percent of federal hospitals had medical school affiliations.

Many of these teaching hospitals are intensely involved in the educational and research processes. They serve as the locus of education for medical and other health professional students and have large biomedical research enterprises. Most of them belong to the Council on Teaching Hospitals (COTH) of the Association of American Medical Colleges. Membership is restricted to hospitals with four approved residency programs in major specialties, affiliation with an accredited medical school, and recommendation for membership by the dean of the school. In 1990,[5] 404 hospitals were nonfederal members of COTH. Sixty-two of them were university-owned and 293 were major affiliates; only 49 were limited affiliates. COTH hospitals are larger hospitals in urban centers, 283 with a bed size greater than 400. All forms of ownership were represented—federal, state, municipal, religious, voluntary, nonvoluntary, for-profit, and not-for-profit.

Of this group of major teaching hospitals, in 1989,[6] there were 123 hospitals that served as the core of AHC. They were either under common ownership with a medical school or were freestanding affiliated hospitals in which the majority of the clinical chiefs of service were department chairs in the affiliated medical school. Approximately half of the medical schools in the United States (61 of 127) had an ownership relation with these hospitals; 23 were jointly owned with private schools and 38 with public schools. The remainder of the AHC hospitals were freestanding, some publicly and some privately owned. In some cases, the institution with the closest relationship to the medical and other health professionals schools was a large multispecialty clinic, for example the Mayo Clinic, instead of a hospital, but in every AHC a relationship exists with some hospital. Only 19 medical schools are not in an AHC coalition, and, even in these cases, they are affiliated in some way with teaching hospitals.

AHC hospitals conduct 79 percent of the GME in the United States. Affiliation of this major educational effort with a medical school does not mean control by the school. Determining the numbers of residents and the content of the training is seldom the province of the medical school administration. Typically, the hospital employs the residents, who act as graduate students of medical departments or disciplines. These residents are under the direct supervision of medical school department chairs, who decide, after consultation with residency review bodies and the hospital administration, the numbers of residents to be recruited into the program and its content. Residents usually have the most intense contact with medical students and are frequently looked upon as very effective teachers. The management of this system by the department and the hospital strengthens the control clinical disciplines have over the content of clinical education for students, increases departmental insularity, and reduces the control of the medical school administration over the clinical education process.

## Contributions to the Health Care System
The contributions of academia to the health care system can be broken into three categories—the educational product of the health professional schools, the research contribution, and the health and medical care provided.

### Education
In 1991,[7] 15,499 students graduated from U.S. medical schools and, in 1990, 1,527[8] from osteopathic schools. The medical school figure is projected to rise to 16,162 by 1995-6. Of those entering medical school in 1990, 69 percent were residents of the state in which the school was located and 38.7 percent were women, a proportion that has stabilized since 1987-88. Minority recruitment has not resulted in major increases in black, native american, or Hispanic students, while asian and pacific islander students have increased significantly. Because of low attrition rates, graduating classes during the next four years can be expected to have the same composition of women and minorities as those presently enrolled.

AHCs are the major supplier of physicians for the United States but produce only a fraction of the national output of nurses and other health professionals. This is not always realized by the public, which often looks to AHCs for solutions to all health manpower problems.

The other critical educational function of academia and AHCs is GME. As of January 1, 1991,[9] there were 82,902 residents in 6,938 programs of residency training in the 1,235[10] teaching hospitals and approximately 340 other institutions offering approved residency training. There were 7,000 more first-year positions available than there were graduates of U.S. medical schools; 22,468 first-year positions were offered for 15,500 U.S. graduates. Many of these unfilled positions went to foreign medical school graduates, now called international medical graduates (IMGs). The term IMG includes U.S. citizens graduating from foreign schools. Although there was a decrease of 3 percent of IMGs in U.S. residencies from 1980 to 1985, there was an increase of 18 percent from 1985 to 1990. This increase is mostly the result of a jump of 31.6 percent in IMGs filling first-year positions.

During that year, the number of IMGs who were not citizens rose 63.4 percent, while U.S. citizens decreased 14.9 percent. The other dramatic increase was in the number of osteopathic graduates seeking training in accredited GME programs. This increase was 265 percent from 1980 to 1990. Thus, residency training positions, increasingly in family medicine, general medicine, and general pediatrics, not filled by graduating physicians from U.S. medical and osteopathic schools are being filled with rising numbers of IMGs, mostly exchange visitors from other countries.

### Research

The research output of academia is difficult to measure. Medical schools are major contributors to the national research effort. They had revenues totaling $4.7 billion in 1989-90 from grants and contracts.[11] This is about 50 percent of the approximately $9 billion national expenditure on biomedical research.[12] Revenue for research is surpassed only by service revenue as a source of support for medical schools. In 1988, 16,586 U.S. physicians, most of them on medical school faculties, reported research as their major full-time activity.[13] At the same time, there were 70,300 full-time faculty members in U.S. schools, most of whom participated part time in research. Obviously, the quantitative research output of academia, as defined by these figures, is substantial. The qualitative nature of this important national resource cannot be accurately measured, but it clearly has become increasingly sophisticated and has produced major enhancements in the pharmacopeia and biotechnology of medicine. Much less of the effort has been quantitative research in health services.

### Health and Medical Care

The health and medical care provided by academia is also difficult to quantify. Faculty members of medical schools in AHCs are usually grouped into corporate entities called practice plans (see Chapter 3). The mission of these plans is to provide broad support to the academic enterprise and to "provide a mechanism for organizing and managing the clinical practice of faculty members consistent with the mission of the academic medical center."[14] Usually, full-time faculty are required to belong to these plans. Most are organized as not-for-profit entities.[15] Members provide a significant amount of the complex care in the United States as the staff of AHC teaching hospitals.

The service outputs of teaching hospitals are an important fraction of the health care in the United States. In 1987, COTH members, constituting only 6 percent of all hospitals, accounted for 23 percent of admissions, 25 percent of births, 28 percent of outpatient visits, and 20 percent of the emergency visits in all short-term, nonfederal hospitals.[16] They were the major providers of complex specialized care: 55 percent of all organ transplant capabilities, 51 percent of hospital-based genetic screening, and 29 percent of hospital-based MRI facilities. They also were major caretakers of the poor, with 21 percent of the short-stay beds, but 32 percent of Medicaid patient days. In 1987, they wrote off 59 percent of the charity care ($2.06 billion) performed by short-term, nonfederal hospitals.

## Basis for Governance Relationships

As has been described, the academic system is a heterogeneous group of entities, often loosely organized, with few similar features, and at different locations. Each of the components of the system is difficult to define, and the organizations that make up the system exhibit many kinds of governance. Relationships are complex and changing. The system of management and control is variable. Despite this complexity, the output of the system is an essential part of the health care delivery system. Academia comprises loose coalitions of powerful institutions, without clear strategic plans or strong direction. Rarely can these institutions give a clear response to public concerns engendered by the importance of their outputs. Any attempt to improve this situation demands that thought be given to the complex governance relationships within academia, particularly in the AHC.

## Governance Relationships
Major controlling forces in the AHC are university administration, AHC administration, medical school administration, and administration of its clinical departments, faculty practice plan, and teaching hospital. In all public and many private universities, federal, state, and community governments also exert control through regulations and resource allocation. Professional schools other than the medical school play a limited role in governance.

## University
University administration is an important force in the governance of AHCs and their medical schools, but, in recent years, this control has eased. Often, components of the AHC are looked upon as sources of major problems for the university. (an example of this attitude is the oft-told story of the university president who, after his death, knew he was in Hell because there were two medical schools.) University boards, potentially important forces in the AHC, have broader concerns, even though in health universities their control may be much more focused. Community leaders and citizens represented on these boards often are not completely aware of the complex nature of the organization and are reluctant to exert their power. As a result, the university administration usually delegates governance of this complex organization to a chief executive officer, often a vice president for health affairs, especially when it owns the teaching hospital. It is only through this layered administration that state and community legislators and leaders, and members of the boards of universities and hospitals, may exert policy control. In state schools, this often leads legislators to feel frustrated in their ability to influence AHC policy and to turn to the appropriations process to exert control. Because of its relative isolation and the large revenue contribution the AHC makes to the central university budget, many AHCs have become almost independent of their parent universities.[17]

## Medical School
As pointed out by Wilson and McLaughlin in their excellent 1984 review of leadership and management in academic medicine,[18] the medical school is difficult to define. Its essence is its faculty members. Where they meet with students is where the educational function of the school takes place, in the clinical years often in the affiliated teaching hospitals. Thus, the school is not a specific location but is defined as a faculty with the core mission of educating medical students.

Clinical faculty members view their responsibility as providing services, in addition to creating new knowledge and transmitting knowledge to students. These faculty members are often not able to satisfy the requirements of traditional tenure appointments because of the demands of their role. This has led to special nontenure appointments in many medical schools, often viewed as less prestigious than tenure but easier to obtain. As a result, faculty numbers have increased 17 percent between 1986-87 and 1990-91,[19] while the number of medical students decreased 2 percent. Clearly, faculty members are needed for more than the educational program. This rapid growth in numbers and the lack of clear definition of the role of clinical faculty is a difficult problem for the traditional medical school and university and has become a source of tension within schools and universities.

Ambiguity of definition is only one of the organizational problems of a medical school. Most deans do not have a management relationship with the faculty that is typical of CEOs in other environments. Growth in the size of the AHC; multiple sources of revenue not under medical school control, particularly for research and from provision of services, including increasing amounts from the hospital; and control of departmental curriculum by faculty members are major factors in the weakening of this role. In addition, the large GME enterprise is almost exclusively a hospital and departmental activity, and other graduate students, also sponsored by departments, may be overseen by graduate or other schools.

Despite these diminished powers, the dean is the traditional leader of the faculty. Prior to World War II, this role had great prestige in the medical school. Though the powers of the dean have been reduced, control of medical school funds, department space budgets, and appointment power of the chairs leave considerable residual power in the position. These powers and the traditional credibility of the office make creative use of the office for leadership of the institution possible.

Department organization, particularly in clinical departments, is a dominant feature of medical schools. The chair usually has the powerful role of chief of hospital service, chair of the medical school department, and leader of the department practice plan. Department faculty feel responsible for curriculum in the discipline and often have an important role in initiation of appointment and promotion of department faculty to be acted on by the chair. They and the chair often determine department budgets for research and teaching to be submitted to the dean. Department practice plans often have management responsibility for department service functions. These key endeavors have produced a tightly knit department structure that is clearly the key unit of the medical school and the AHC.

### Faculty Practice Plans

Faculty practice plans (FPP) have been increasingly important sources of revenue for medical schools and teaching hospitals. In a 1991 study by the Association of American Medical Colleges,[20] FPP were described as being organized as either not-for-profit corporations, charitable trusts, foundations, partnerships, or professional corporations. These entities are exempt from most federal, state, and local taxes. In private schools, they are more often organized within the school (74 percent); in public schools, they are more often outside of the school (57 percent). The reason for this difference appears to be the desire in public schools to lessen government control. Plans attempt to straddle the line between independence and participation in the AHC and, like chameleons, can assume either image as necessity dictates. This adaptability is present in almost every plan, even when they have different structures, some strictly departmental, others as a single organization of disciplines.

Faculty practice plans have strong faculty governance systems. Usually, there is a large governing board with strong physician leadership. Though deans are often members of the plans (86 percent of the plans studied by AAMC), they and vice presidents for health affairs, university officials, and hospital CEOs who are occasionally members are rarely controlling forces. The boards, on the other hand, exert strong control over billing systems, strategic planning, and marketing. Fee schedule setting is the only function that is more likely to be a department or discipline responsibility. Frequently, a single faculty physician, elected as chair of the board, assumes the powerful role of director of the plan.

Faculty practice plans have contributed a steadily rising proportion of total revenues for medical schools. These revenues were 14.5 percent of the total in 1981-1982 and 27 percent of the total in 1988-1989.[20] In almost all plans there is a "dean's tax" on revenues that varies from 2 to 18 percent. In most cases, this money is allocated to the dean for medical school development. Of course, most service revenue goes to direct support of faculty income, as decided by the plan and departments, often under guidelines set by the department and approved by the dean. Frequently, a nearly equal amount is set aside for development of the department, further strengthening department autonomy.

Faculty practice plans add significant complexity to the management of the AHC by enhancing the controlling force of the clinical faculty and its departments. Plans have special power in hospital affairs, where the medical school administration is often a mendicant.

## Teaching Hospitals

Teaching hospitals add yet another degree of intricacy to the governance structure of the AHC. COTH hospitals add education of health professionals and clinical research to their mission of patient service. They are, by themselves, large, complex organizations[16] usually located in urban areas. In 1989, they employed 29 percent of all U.S. registered nurses and 61 percent of all salaried physicians and dentists working in short-term nonfederal hospitals. They trained 79 percent of the residents in U.S. hospitals. Their staffs are almost always members of the FPP of the clinical departments of the medical school.

As has been described, teaching hospitals exhibit variable ownership relationships with the medical school and the university. Typically, the they are not-for-profit, often with their origins as indigent care institutions. They often have boards of trustees that are separate from those of the university/medical school. The director of the university hospital, most commonly a trained manager, is faced with the difficult role of ensuring that the educational and research missions are consonant with patient services. This administration must strive to keep the hospital a competitive health care provider in the community, while offering large amounts of charity care, maintaining a technologically advanced physical facility, maintaining a large GME program, and providing a locus for education of medical and other health professional students.

AHC hospitals are undergoing change. As pointed out by Munson and D'Aunno in their study of university hospitals,[21] in some cases divestiture of a university hospital from the parent medical school/university is being considered. Some of the most successful AHC hospitals in the United States are owned separately from associated medical schools.

In 1946, another group of important hospitals began to join the list of AHCs.[22] Following World War II, there was an acute shortage of physicians in Veterans

## Table 1. Academic Health Organizations and Missions[*]

| | |
|---|---|
| University<br>Health/Medical University | Education.<br>Research.<br>Public Service. |
| Academic Health Center | Coordination of Units.<br>Relations with University.<br>Relations with Public. |
| Medical School | Medical Student Education.<br>Biomedical Research. |
| Clinical Department | Graduate Medical Education.<br>Patient Care.<br>Applied Biomedical Research.<br>Medical Student Education. |
| Health Related Professional School | Education of Other Health Professionals.<br>Applied Research. |
| Faculty Practice Plan | Bill and Collect for Patient Services.<br>Mechanism to Recruit, Retain and<br>    Compensate Faculty Physicians.<br>Supply Revenue to Support Academic<br>    Programs. |
| Teaching Hospitals<br>    Nonfederal<br>    Federal | Patient Care.<br>Graduate Medical Education.<br>Medical Student Education.<br>Health Professional Education.<br>Research. |

[*] Missions are arranged in order of organizational priority.

Administration (VA) hospitals. AHCs were a potential source of these physicians. The result was Public Law 79-293 and the now well-known VA Policy Memorandum No. 2, which stated that, in affiliation with medical schools, while the VA would retain full responsibility for the care of patients, including professional treatment, the school of medicine would accept responsibility for all graduate education and training. In FY 1989, 103 of 126 medical schools were affiliated with one or more VA facilities. Some of these include the VA hospital as an integral part of the AHC. Indeed, as a result of the Health Manpower Training Act of 1972, five new state medical schools to be affiliated with VA hospitals were established. Federal funds were also provided to expand class size in other medical schools with VA affiliations.

The governance of VA hospitals is through the federal Department of

## Table 2. Classes of Teaching Hospitals

| Hospital Type | Educational Functions Relationships | Number of Hospitals[1] |
|---|---|---|
| Community Hospital | Several Programs of GME. | 963 |
| Affiliated Hospital | Affiliated with Medical School with/without GME. | 1054 |
| Member, Council of Teaching Hospitals (COTH) | Four specified[2] residencies. Affiliated with Medical School. Accredited by LCME.[3] Recommendation of Dean. | 404 |
| Veterans Hospitals (COTH members) | GME. Medical Student Education. | 70 |
| Academic Health Center Hospitals | A COTH Hospital with Chiefs of Service as Medical School Department Heads or Common Ownership with Medical School. | 123 |

1. Numbers of hospitals are 1989 or 1990 data. Other than VA hospitals, numbers are for short-term, nonfederal hospitals.
2. Four programs of GME, with at least two from family practice, internal medicine, obstetrics/gynecology, pediatrics, psychiatry, or surgery.
3. Liaison Committee on Medical Education, the accrediting body for medical schools.

Veterans Affairs. At the university level, there is a dean's committee that coordinates activities between the partners and approves appointments. The most intense management interest of the medical school is at the level of department chair. Variable mutual relationships are developed by medical school departments with VA departments and administration. GME and research programs are most related at this level. The AHC has limited control of these arrangements. While the farsighted alliance of the VA and academia has been a boon, it has also added another degree of complexity to the management of AHCs.

The changes now occurring in the VA system—dwindling numbers of veterans eligible for service, increasing lengths of stay, aging of U.S. veterans, and decreasing federal resources—have led to new initiatives in long-term care, geriatrics, and rehabilitation and even recommendation that the VA system be opened to nonveterans in certain underserved communities, a move that will have an impact on AHCs.

## Summary
Academia, as the word is used in health education, consists of a number of organizations (table 1, page 8) with various missions. Each of these organizations has a CEO. Only in the case of teaching hospitals is there a high probability that the CEO has had formal training in management. There is great variability in the

power relationships between the units in different institutions. In aggregate, these organizations produce a significant number of physicians and other health professionals, perform much of the country's graduate medical education and clinical research, and provide a significant amount of the complex medical care in the United States.

Teaching hospitals are the main contact point of academia with the health care system. They can be arranged into several classes (table 2, page 9). It is through these hospitals that academic institutions provide direct health and medical care. A small number of them, largely academic health center hospitals, are the sites of much of the complex health and medical care performed, much of the GME, and most clinical medical student teaching done in academia. Thus, this relatively small number of AHCs exert considerable influence on the health care system. These consortia, centered on a medical school and one or more teaching hospitals staffed by faculty of the medical school, have as their essential units clinical departments with considerable power to generate revenue resulting from the provision of highly complex medical care. This has resulted in the hiring of larger numbers of faculty than needed to satisfy the educational mission. When grouped into faculty practice plans, these faculty have enhanced revenue generation and have strengthened the role of their departments as the fundamental units of the AHC and the medical school.

Academia is faced with growing, important, and complex problems. Medical student education is shifting to the more costly ambulatory environment during a period when resources for education are decreasing. National concern grows about health care costs, and reductions seem imminent in federal subsidization of GME. Shortages and maldistribution of primary care physicians have become an important national issue, a problem not suitable for solution in the AHC, and the trend toward managed health care has placed AHC faculty and hospitals in tough competition with the private sector.

Despite the complex nature of the relationship of academia to the health care delivery system, its contribution to the education of professionals, application of research, and provision of services for the people have been immense. New challenges, requiring new efforts, must be faced by academia if the health care system is to maintain its level of contribution to U.S. citizens' health. Clearly, the management of academic institutions will be an important ingredient in the success of these efforts.

## References

1. Jonas, H., and others. "Educational Programs in U.S. Medical Schools." *JAMA* 266(7):913-20, Aug. 21, 1991.

2. Ludmerer, K. *Learning to Heal: The Development of American Medical Education.* New York, N.Y.: Basic Books, Inc., 1985.

3. Starr, P. *The Social Transformation of American Medicine.* New York, N.Y.: Basic Books, Inc., 1982.

4. *AHA Hospital Statistics.* Chicago, Ill.: American Hospital Association, 1990, p. 202, table 10A.

5. *AAMC Data Book, Statistical Information Related to Medical Education.* Washington, D.C.: Association of American Medical Colleges, May 1990, table G8.

6. AAMC listing of academic health center hospitals, May 24, 1989.

7. Jonas, H., and others. *Op. cit.*, p. 916.

8. *1991 Yearbook and Directory of Osteopathic Physicians.* Chicago, Ill.: American Osteopathic Association, 1991, p. 519.

9. Rowley, B., and others. "Selected Characteristics of Graduate Medical Education in the United States." *JAMA* 266(7):933-43, Aug. 21, 1991.

10. *AHA Hospital Statistics.* Chicago, Ill.: American Hospital Association, 1991, p. 202, table 10A.

11. Jolin, L., and others. "U.S. Medical School Finances." *JAMA* 266(7):985-90, Aug. 21, 1991.

12. U.S. Bureau of the Census. *Statistical Abstract of the United States: 1991.* 111th Edition. Washington, D.C.: U.S. Government Printing Office, 1991, p. 590.

13. *AAMC Data Book, Statistical Information Related to Medical Education.* Washington, D.C.: Association of American Medical Colleges, May 1990, table J1.

14. *Faculty Practice Plans: The Organization and Characteristics of Academic Medical Practice.* Washington, D.C.: Association of American Medical Colleges, 1991.

15. *Ibid*, p. 10, figure 3.

16. *Teaching Hospitals: Multiple Roles, Distinctive Characteristics.* Chusid, J., Editor. Washington, D.C.: Association of American Medical Colleges, July 1989.

17. Ginzberg, E. *The Medical Triangle. Physicians, Politicians, and the Public.* Cambridge, Mass.: Harvard University Press, 1990, p. 61.

18. Wilson, M., and McLaughlin, C. *Leadership and Management in Academic Medicine.* San Francisco, Calif.: Jossey-Bass Publishers, 1984.

19. Jonas, H. *Op. cit.*, p. 914.

20. *Faculty Practice Plans.* Washington, D.C.: Association of American Medical Colleges, 1991, p. 21.

21. Munson, F., and D'Aunno, T. *The University Hospital in the Academic Health Center: Finding the Right Relationship.* Volumes I and II. Washington, D.C.: Association of American Medical Colleges, 1987.

22. *The Partnership: VA Hospitals and Graduate Medical Education.* Washington, D.C.: Association of American Medical Colleges, June 1990.

*Charles C. Lobeck, MD, is Professor Emeritus, Pediatrics and Preventive Medicine, Programs in Health Management, University of Wisconsin Medical School, Madison, Wisconsin.*

# Chapter 2

# The Teaching, Research, and Clinical Triad

*by Mahendr S. Kochar, MD, MS, MBA*

# The Overall Mission

The overall mission of an Academic Health Center (AHC) is to provide cutting edge tertiary and quaternary health care in a milieu of education and research. From a medical school's point of view, the primary mission of an AHC is to provide undergraduate medical education to its students while simultaneously conducting research and training residents and fellows to become specialists. Many of the medical school's research laboratories are located in the hospital, and some research-oriented faculty members may believe that the primary mission of the AHC is medical research. They may say that patients are needed to provide "clinical material" for this effort and that the patient care is a byproduct of education and research and not the main purpose of an academic hospital. For the managers of AHCs, it is often a challenge to maintain a balance between these multiple missions.[1]

## External Influences

The external forces influencing policy and administration in AHCs are government, private and professional groups, and the community. They include government at all levels, professional organizations, private foundations, national voluntary health organizations, regional and local community interests, physicians, and hospitals. Local governments and the public often look upon the AHC as a source of charity care to the uninsured, the indigent, and critically wounded patients. They may not be concerned about how the AHC is funded and take it for granted that the hospital will somehow always be there to provide care to those who cannot afford it.

The social contract between AHCs and society requires them to prepare physicians for practice, to advance medicine by developing new knowledge, and to demonstrate optimum use of existing and new knowledge by providing health services to the public. This broad set of social obligations is carried out through a number of distinct activities or programs that are dictated by strong forces outside the centers as well as within them. These are not always mutually supportive and, indeed, may conflict with each other. This lack of unity and its overall social purpose distinguish the AHC from other large organizations in the corporate world.[1]

## The Teaching Mission

Undergraduate medical education of students in their second, third, and fourth years of medical school takes place primarily in academic hospitals. During the junior (third) year, students in most medical schools undergo eight-week "clerkships" in medicine, surgery, obstetrics and gynecology, pediatrics, psychiatry, and ambulatory care. During the senior (fourth) year, they receive training in such specialties of medicine as ophthalmology, orthopedics, ENT, etc. and, at most medical schools, can take up to six months of electives, depending on their interests. Much of this training is imparted by residents who are only a year or two senior to the students.

### Graduate Medical Education

Graduate medical education (GME) is a very important mission of an AHC. Although there are community teaching hospitals that are unaffiliated or only loosely affiliated with medical schools and provide housestaff training, for the past 20 years, AHC hospitals have increased their share of GME. Part of the reason for this is the need to have more housestaff to assist with the increasingly complex and technology-dependent tertiary and quaternary care that these hospitals provide. The housestaff is often required to spend long hours providing service to patients, which cuts into the time needed for didactic education. There has been media and public criticism of the AHC for this reason and some have questioned the quality of care provided by the "tired" housestaff. AHC hospitals are very sensitive to this issue, and many are addressing it by hiring physician extenders to do more routine tasks, such as insertion of intravenous needles and drawing of blood, so that the housestaff can rest at night.

Housestaff training is an opportunity to learn by doing. This requires that residents be given increasing responsibility commensurate with their training. Supervision by the faculty is an integral part of the housestaff training. Medicare reimburses the hospitals for the residents' salaries and faculty supervision in the form of direct medical education costs. The indirect medical education adjustment, which is currently reimbursed by Medicare at the rate of 7.4 percent of the direct cost, was added to the Medicare Prospective Payment System in recognition of the specialized services and treatment programs made available to severely ill patients at teaching institutions and the additional costs associated with the teaching of residents.

The AHC needs space—office space, conference rooms, auditoriums, sleeping quarters for the housestaff, libraries, etc.—dedicated to teaching and learning. These needs add to the cost of running an AHC.

Prior to the introduction of Medicare in 1965, much of clinical teaching was performed by practicing physicians who held clinical appointments in medical school departments and were not compensated for their teaching efforts. With the ability to bill insurance companies for physician services, the number of full-time faculty members in medical schools has skyrocketed, and almost all the teaching is now done by paid faculty members. In recent years, in order to provide increasing volume and intensity of care to AHC patients, this number continues to rise.

### Rewards of Teaching

To succeed as an academic physician, one is expected to be a "triple-threat," demonstrating excellence in clinical work, teaching, and research. Most AHCs have come to realize that it is no longer possible for every faculty member to be a triple-threat and that one should be satisfied with attaining excellence in one or, at the most, two of the three areas.[2] This has caused many medical schools to introduce a dual-track promotion system—one track for physicians who excel in research and the other for those who excel in teaching and clinical work. At some of the medical schools, tenure is denied to those in the clinician-educator track. If the word "clinical" is used in the title of the faculty member in the clinician-educator track, it creates an impression of second-class citizenship and may cause conflict among faculty members.

Rewarding teaching is not easy. Teaching does not generate funds, unless it is a byproduct of patient care. As stated before, university promotion committees also do not readily recognize teaching for promotion and tenure purposes.[3] Awards for excellence in teaching by students and residents can be given to only a handful of individuals. Some of the medical schools have formed "teaching scholar societies" and recognize excellence in teaching by awarding membership in these societies. The role of these societies in the AHC is ambiguous, as they often exist outside the mainstream of faculty governance.

## The Research Mission

Without research, it is difficult, if not impossible, to educate and train physicians to provide modern, scientifically based health care. Research helps ensure that the medical faculty is on the frontier of new knowledge and can apply it readily in the care of patients, thus implementing and demonstrating its value without undue delay.

### Research Support

In Western European countries, national research policy has continued to rely heavily on research institutes and centers. While many of the centers and institutes have some affiliation with universities and their medical schools, they are distinct entities whose responsibilities are very clear. For example, in Great Britain, the research staff is paid directly by the Medical Research Council (MRC).[4] In the United States, most biomedical research is done at AHCs, and freestanding research institutions or centers are the exception. Research supported by the National Institutes of Health (NIH) and the National Science Foundation has been the largest single factor responsible for the substantial growth in medical school faculties since World War II in the United States.

Large national voluntary agencies interested in particular health problems also create opportunities for AHCs by supporting research and, on occasion, demonstrations of more effective and comprehensive care. Larger organizations, such as the American Heart Association and the American Cancer Society, obtain contributions from community campaigns that are used to support research, public education, and demonstrations of improved care for patients. Their policies are determined jointly by lay persons interested in particular health problems and by professional experts. While their financial capabilities are limited, they influence AHCs by their decisions about what lines of research and what types of demonstrations of health care they will support.

Some new procedures, when they first become available, are not reimbursed by Medicare and the insurance companies, as they are considered experimental. As these procedures become well established and their efficacy in preventing death and increasing survival is demonstrated, insurance companies start to reimburse physicians as well as hospitals for them. However, there is a period during which there are no research funds to support these procedures and hospitals are not reimbursed. This can pose a serious problem for hospitals, as these expenses can be very large.

## Rewards of Research

Support for research by the federal government and other outside sources represents roughly one-quarter of the budgets of medical schools. All of this research is performed by members of the faculty who have academic tenure or are striving for it. At a time when national support for research is stable or declining, faculty members are under persistent pressure to compete successfully for continued and enlarged financial support. Research capacity, proven or expected, is the single most crucial factor in evaluating the suitability of individuals for faculty appointment and promotion. It is assumed that there is always a direct positive relationship between an increasing amount of productive research in the AHC and the quality of the education and patient care it provides. Faculty members perceive that their research effort is critical to their status on the faculty, as outside support for their research often provides all or part of their salary and that of their close colleagues and assistants. Best faculty members often inevitably believe that their time for research must be jealously guarded and tend to relegate the care of patients and the teaching of medical students and residents to a less important position. Many department heads claim that all of their faculty members are equally interested in research, patient care, and teaching and that they expect all faculty members of clinical departments to behave that way.

## Nature of Research

Most of the research performed at an AHC is overwhelmingly biomedical in nature. The great progress made in biomedical research has provided new insights into the biological mechanisms of disease and has led to new modes of diagnosis and treatment. It has also fostered the development of new technology that adds precision to medical care and has opened up new areas of investigation. As a consequence of current research priorities, medical education inevitably focuses predominantly on organic factors in health and disease processes. The service, teaching, and research activities undertaken to meet challenging societal needs are generally at the periphery of the AHC's interests rather than at its core and rarely compete successfully with traditional, entrenched faculty interests. Social science research in health has been only minimally developed, and then primarily in relation to mental health.

## Research Space

Space is almost always at a premium in AHCs. Research requires laboratory, office, and conference room space. Faculty members with larger research grants need and expect more space. Research space can also become a prestige issue. Solomon has proposed a mathematical formula for allocating research space.[5] Even if a faculty member's research grant is not renewed, he or she needs to continue research to remain competitive while reapplying for grants. During this interim period, the AHC has to pick up not only salaries but also the cost of space.

## The Clinical Service

It is service to patients that generates funds for the hospitals, but the academic hospital often has uninsured and indigent patients referred to it by practicing physicians as well as by community hospitals, even if these patients do not require sophisticated tertiary and quaternary care. Current societal problems, such as violence, AIDs, drug abuse, hopelessness, and drunk driving, generate seriously ill or injured patients who often do not have insurance and who are brought to AHCs because community hospitals shun them. Although these cases provide excellent experience and teaching for students and housestaff, their care often goes unreimbursed.[6]

Increasing numbers of Americans are enrolling in health maintenance organizations (HMOs) for their health care, but HMOs generally avoid doing business with academic hospitals because of their high expenses, as controlling costs is important to the success of any managed care plan. This has caused some AHCs to start their own HMOs. Practicing physicians often believe that academic hospitals and faculty physicians should simply be content with taking care of the indigent and uninsured patients. On the other hand, AHCs and their faculties feel that community hospitals should refer all patients for tertiary and quaternary care to AHCs. This often leads to a "town-gown" conflict that can sometimes be very difficult to resolve.

In order to increase their market shares, AHCs are adopting various strategies.[7] Some have entered into networking relationships with community hospitals, and their full-time faculty members on a regular basis hold clinics in these hospitals. As a result, every patient referred to the AHC does not need to go to the AHC and can be taken care of in the community hospital where the patient's physician practices and near where the patient lives. Only patients requiring tertiary or quaternary care are brought to the AHC for admission.

### Ambulatory Care

Increasing numbers of AHCs have found it necessary to provide facilities where students and housestaff can be trained in ambulatory medicine. With the development of noninvasive diagnostic technology, the public's wish to avoid hospitalization, and the insurance industry's reluctance to pay for in-hospital care when outpatient care suffices, ambulatory care has in recent years gained a great deal of momentum. As more community hospitals have entered the arena of tertiary and even quaternary care and as referrals of insured patients to academic hospitals has declined, it has been necessary for AHCs to develop their own primary care systems from which patients can be referred for not only teaching and research purposes but also for revenue. The ambulatory care centers, by themselves, rarely generate profit for the AHCs. The opening of an ambulatory clinic by the AHC away from the parent AHC is often viewed by community physicians as a threat to the size of their practices. This can further aggravate the "town and gown" conflict, making it quite severe.

## Governance

In the typical business corporation, the hierarchy of control is much clearer than it is in an AHC. While professional and technical expertise among the corporation's employees is sought when needed, the power of decision making rests with the top management of the corporation. This provides the typical corporate structure, with clear and effective means to examine its goals and procedures in the face of new problems or opportunities, and gives a great deal of flexibility in organizing activities. Effective administration of the AHC hospital calls for consistent, strong competence and clearly recognized authority as it develops and operates its services while providing opportunities for education and research. The challenge and requirements of AHC governance are essentially the same whether it is freestanding or part of a public or private university.

### Role of the Chair

The hospital medical staff either exclusively or predominantly comprises the full-time faculty of the clinical departments of the medical school that owns the AHC or with which the AHC hospital is affiliated. Department heads at the medical school are also department heads at the hospital. The clinical chairs usually behave as though the medical school and the hospital are one organization. Department chairs are usually appointed because of their demonstrated competence as scientists.[8] Many want to continue their own research and try to guard their time for this purpose. However, not all have the leadership qualities needed to form people of diverse backgrounds and interests into a team to function in an optimum fashion.[9]

All medical school departments fund a large portion of their expenditures—not uncommonly more than one-half and sometimes more than two-thirds—from external sources for special projects and programs and, in the case of clinical departments, from fees for patient care. They tend to view these funds, which they have "generated," as "belonging" solely to them and not available for other school programs. These externally funded activities need space and supporting services, requiring institutional concurrence and support of the medical school and the hospitals, thus influencing the priorities of these institutions. To meet these needs, the faculty, in its many discrete parts, believes it should have a dominant role in policy making and management. Intrafaculty competition and rivalries among faculty groups have increased. Within departments, although there is usually an atmosphere of collegiality, the chair has a great deal of authority and generally makes the final decision. In larger departments that are organized into sizable subspecialty units, competing priorities present special problems for the chair.

### Role of the Faculty

Essentially, the top administration of the AHC operates as a loose conglomeration of independent units. It enfranchises groups of faculty members to carry out their professional tasks as virtually independent units. This independence exists not only because of the university framework but also because of the rapid and massive growth of the centers as collections of distinct, highly specialized activities, discretely financed through faculty initiatives, including fees for clinical services. Because faculty members develop their status in academia because of their professional performance, including their ability to "get grants," they naturally expect a large voice in policy making. At a minimum, they expect the administration to expedite their work by giving it the highest priority and providing space and the necessary supporting services. In the present period of financial constraints, they expect the administration to find additional funds or to reallocate existing institutional funds to maintain their efforts, if not to facilitate their growth.[10] A "we/they" viewpoint prevails within most centers: "We," the faculty, are working hard, doing excellent work in the eyes of our peers, while "they," the administration, doesn't really appreciate how important it is and doesn't help enough.

### Role of the Dean

Many faculty members believe that the dean should serve their needs as they see them and that the dean's role is to carry out the majority decisions of faculty committees. A less prevalent view is that the dean, having earned the trust and support of the faculty, should, after consultation, have the authority to use his or her best judgment. Most faculty members are uncertain which of these patterns of governance is best.

The authority and responsibility of not only the dean vis-a-vis the faculty but also that of the hospital administrator vis-a-vis the medical staff are ambiguous at best.[11] Because most decisions affecting programs and activities are made at the departmental and subdepartmental level, it is difficult for the institution to give the long-term institutional implications of those decisions timely, consistent, and effective attention. People outside the institution push for intraorganizational change, and, simultaneously, there are pressures from the inside to maintain the status quo and insulate the organization from external influences. In the face of shrinking funds and persistent external and internal pressure, the current form of governance tends to foster short-term solutions instead of the long-term planning that is needed. Highly skilled professionals accustomed to autonomy and independence do not take well to administrators, even when they share a common background in terms of basic scientific medical training.

### Challenge to Administrators

AHC administrators face one of the most complex administrative tasks. They are managing highly technical and diverse research enterprises. They seek to organize this research so that those who conduct it contribute their knowledge to graduate and postgraduate medical instruction and to the medical services of teaching hospitals. They have to coordinate the activities of highly trained specialists who take a dim view of administration. In addition, AHCs face a heightened expectation of accountability and cost-effectiveness.

Academic hospitals must function within the framework of the overall national reimbursement and delivery system and at the same time fit the ways of medical schools and faculty physicians. Some believe that the AHC must take responsibility for the delivery of the full range of medical care so that, while carrying out its tertiary care functions, it gives creative attention to primary and secondary care and to the optimum relationship between all three levels of care. It must become involved in the full range of health problems in their service area.

## Acknowledgement

I found the book *The Sick Citadel*, by Irving J. Lewis and Cecil G. Sheps, to be a particularly useful source of information in writing this chapter and have drawn on it extensively. I recommend it highly to those interested in learning more about the conflicts and the challenges facing academic health centers. Although the book was written a decade ago, the problems facing AHCs that are mentioned in the book have not gone away; if anything, they have grown, and new ones have been added. The book is referenced below.

# References

1. Lewis, I., and Sheps, C. *The Sick Citadel.* Cambridge, Mass.: Oelgeschlager, Gunn, and Hain, 1983.

2. Mirvis, D. "Physicians in Organizations: Dilemma of the Academic VA Staff Physician." *Archives of Internal Medicine* 150(8):1621-3, Aug. 1990.

3. Glaser, R. "The Academic Recognition of Clinical Teachers." *Phases of AOA Honorary Medical Society* 52(1):33, Winter 1989.

4. Booth, C. "The National Health Service, the Universities, and the Research Council: The Future of Academic Medicine." *British Medical Journal* 296(6633):1382-5, May 14, 1988.

5. Solomon, S., and Tom, S. "Allocating Research Space in the University Medical Center: Use of a Mathematical Formula." *American Journal of Medical Science* 297(1):3-8, Jan. 1989.

6. Davidson, R. "Viewpoint: Academic Medical Centers—It's Time for a Declaration of Values." *Health Care Management Review* 15(2):81-5, Spring 1990.

7. Morris, D. "Winning Strategies for Academic Centers." *Health Care Strategy Management* 6(7):14-6, July 1988.

8. Petersdorf, R., and Wilson, M. "The Four Horsemen of the Apocalypse." *JAMA* 247(8):1153-61, Feb. 26, 1982.

9. Aluise, J., and others. "Administrative Skills for Academic Physicians." *Medical Teacher* 11(2):205-12, 1989.

10. Ehrle, E., and Bennett, J. *Managing the Academic Enterprise. Case Studies for Deans and Provosts.* New York, N.Y.: McMillan, 1988.

11. Wilson, M., and McLaughlin, C. *Leadership and Management in Academic Medicine.* San Francisco, Calif.: Jossey-Bass, 1984.

*Mahendr S. Kochar, MD, MS, MBA, is Executive Director, Medical College of Wisconsin Affiliated Hospitals, Inc.; Associate Dean for Graduate Medical Education and Professor, Departments of Medicine and Pharmacology/ Toxicology, Medical College of Wisconsin; and Associate Chief of Staff for Education and Chief of Hypertension, Zablocki VA Medical Center, Milwaukee, Wisconsin.*

# Chapter 3

# Faculty Practice Plans

*by Sam J. W. Romeo, MD, MBA, FACPE*

The precursor to faculty practice plans (FPPs) was the full-time clinical faculty system that was introduced in the early 20th Century to provide a milieu that would foster clinical research. This plan was developed by preclinical scientists at the Johns Hopkins Medical School, Baltimore, Maryland, and was inaugurated there in 1913 with the financial assistance of the Rockefeller General Education Board.[1] As this model was adopted across the country, clinical faculties at U.S. medical schools complemented their research and educational responsibilities by providing professional medical services to patients. From 1913 through the 1950s the clinical faculty system remained small and unchanged in its mission. A small number of faculty clinicians continued to provide care to indigent patients, with their compensation being provided primarily through the medical schools. Only modest fees were generated by patients.

Faculty practice plans proliferated in the 1960s, with more than 70 percent of current FPPs being developed in that decade.[2] The impetus for the creation of so many FPPs is largely linked to the creation of Medicare and Medicaid in the middle of the decade. Medicare and Medicaid were the first two major innovations in paying for health care since Blue Cross/Blue Shield was established in 1939 in response to the depression. As more Americans became covered by health insurance plans—Medicare, Medicaid, or commercial insurance companies—and sought out health care, medical schools needed to develop practice plans that would effectively manage the billing and collection process resulting from clinical care.

FPPs are therefore commonly defined as an organized arrangement for billing and for distributing revenue according to some agreed upon formula to the medical school departments and individual clinicians providing the care. FPPs provide a mechanism to distribute the revenue generated by the faculty's clinical practice. The 1913 distribution model introduced at Johns Hopkins is known as the full-time plan; faculty members earn a base salary plus income from their clinical practice, usually with a ceiling on earnings. In another full-time distribution model operating within medical school FPPs, faculty members receive only a fixed salary based on academic rank and institutional policy.

To accomplish the tasks of billing, collection, and distribution, in addition to faculty compensation and management of the income stream, FPPs tend to be organized on the basis of a department model, a federal model, or a group model. The departmental model is characterized by department autonomy and has little or no overarching governance or coordination. The department model is the least structured of faculty practice plans. The federal model is characterized by some measure of common governance and by management by an informal advisory committee that decides policies. The group model has a high degree of common governance and has clinical faculty input into policy decisions.

While 74 of 125 medical schools responding to a survey classify themselves as group models, close review of their governance and administrative structures discloses that they are distributed along the spectrum between decentralized department models and centralized group models.[3]

Faculty practice plans operate within 126 medical schools.[3] Whether an FPP operates within a private or a public medical school, all have common characteristics. Although each practice plan will have its own mission statement and objectives, all practice plans have consistent philosophies within their mission statements that guide their management and operation:

■ To encourage superior patient care, teaching, and research.

■ To bill and collect for medical services provided by clinical staff.

■ To provide a mechanism that is consistent with the mission of the medical school for organizing and managing the clinical practice of faculty members.

■ To provide a source of revenue to support the academic programs of the medical school.

■ To ensure that there are a sufficient number and variety of patients for education and research.

Medical schools have struggled historically to maintain their primary focus of training and educating medical students and to conduct research. This focus became more difficult in the 1970s and 1980s, when American taxpayers decided that the public was not the sole beneficiary of the education of a physician.[4] Taxpayers felt that the process of becoming a physician was an individual endeavor with individual benefits. As a result, public subsidy of medical education was severely restricted, while medical schools' role in research continued to expand.

As the cost of a medical education soared, attendance in medical schools could be financed individually only by a very few wealthy students. Lacking public support for education and fearful of government support meaning government control, medical schools turned to research grants to support their scholarly endeavors. These grants enabled medical schools to continue their tradition of educating future doctors while building clinical departments to conduct research. However, federal grants still did not provide sufficient income to guarantee that a medical school would be able to continue its mission of educating future physicians. Additionally, some medical schools were unable to successfully compete for grant money, which severely threatened their solvency.

As revenue sources for education declined and as double-digit inflation elevated the costs associated with government obligations under Medicare and Medicaid to provide health care benefits to those entitled under the law, state and federal legislators began reducing budgets for research. Reduced support for education and research has resulted in FPPs' need to become more organized and efficient.

Faculty practice plans have developed an increasingly prominent and critical role in the income base of medical schools. Indeed, the delivery of health care, in many instances, is seen as a substitute for research and education and grants as the raison d'etre for FPPs within medical schools.

Faculty practice plans will need to forge increasingly important bonds with their communities; with third-party payers, including government; and with managed care systems. FPPs are in the enviable and unique posture of being able to position themselves in the forefront of health care delivery while providing financial stability for the institutions that have nurtured their development. Given the new prominence and promise of FPPs in the organizational structure of medical schools, it is important to understand their design, function, and characteristics.

Because faculty practice plans were developed as a means of managing the income stream generated by medical school physicians and because of the new found reliance medical schools have on their practice plans, efficient day-to-day operations of FPPs is becoming essential. There are multiple models on which medical schools have based their practice plans. However, there are several intrinsic characteristics that are common to all practice plans: governance, organizational structure, billing systems, practice settings, faculty compensation, and the locus for decision making.

It is often said that, if you know one faculty practice plan, you know one faculty practice plan. Using the previous model divisions—group, federal, and department—we will attempt to put order into these variations. All of the models perform five major functions: financial direction, strategic planning, letting of contracts, setting of fees, and general administration (see figure 1, below). Seventy-four medical colleges, in response to a 1990 survey by the Association of American Medical Colleges, indicated these responsibilities belonged to a governing board (group model) or the individual clinical department (department model) or were a function of both the board and the department (federal model).[3]

Because governing boards have such significant roles to play in the group and federal models in the operation of the practice plans, the composition of these boards is critical. Board members must have educational and professional backgrounds that allow them to focus the professional direction of the college and the business acumen of a large corporate CEO. Most governing boards are health care

## Figure 1. Vested Policy Making Authority

| Function | Group Model | Department Model | Federal Model | No Response |
|---|---|---|---|---|
| Financial | 26 | 14 | 27 | 7 |
| Strategic Planning | 21 | 16 | 31 | 6 |
| Contracts | 24 | 8 | 30 | 12 |
| Fees | 8 | 44 | 14 | 38 |
| General Admission | 25 | 15 | 27 | 7 |

driven and have strong physician representation. Other members of a governing board are typically a hospital CEO; a university representative; and, in a few instances, a community representative. Governing boards provide the expertise and experience through which a practice plan is able to accomplish the goals, objectives, and mission of both the FPP and the medical school.

Because faculty participation is essential to the financial stability of medical schools, participation in practice plans is mandatory in 94 percent of the 74 medical schools surveyed in the 1990 AAMC report.[3] This 94 percent mandatory participation relates to full-time faculty staff. Mandatory participation in practice plans is required 50 percent of the time for part-time faculty.

Directly correlated to mandatory participation in the faculty practice plan is faculty compensation. In medical schools in which faculty practice plans are based on the full-time model, 66 percent of the schools provide a base salary, with clinical faculty supplementing their salaries through clinical practice with a ceiling limit. This structure provides an economic incentive for physicians, while maintaining an income stream for the medical school.

Faculty paychecks for work performed for FPPs are generated by diverse pay agents. Faculty paychecks are generated from the employing university as the pay agent for faculty in 45 percent of practice plans. A single paycheck from the university and the plan as a joint pay agent for faculty is the case in 2 percent of practice plans, and two paychecks, one from the university and one from the plan, each a pay agent for faculty, is the case in 41 percent of the FPPs. Twelve percent of the medical schools did not identify a pay agent for their faculties.[3]

Another important component of practice plans is legal structure (see figure 2, below). Some practice plans are organized as separate associations or corporations outside the medical school system, while others are organized within the school

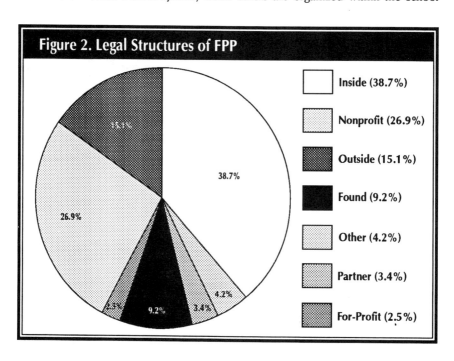

**Figure 2. Legal Structures of FPP**

Inside (38.7%)

Nonprofit (26.9%)

Outside (15.1%)

Found (9.2%)

Other (4.2%)

Partner (3.4%)

For-Profit (2.5%)

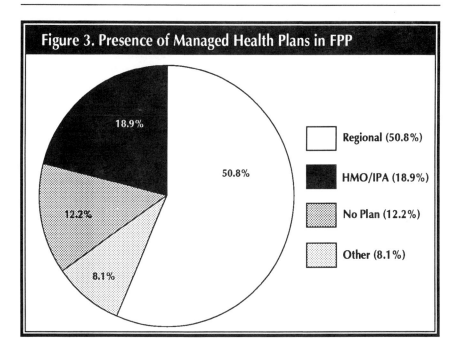

Figure 3. Presence of Managed Health Plans in FPP

Regional (50.8%)

HMO/IPA (18.9%)

No Plan (12.2%)

Other (8.1%)

system. Some practice plans are organized as for-profit entities, others as not-for-profit. Still others have the structure of a foundation or partnership. Some medical schools have practice plans with two or more structures.

Because the formation of practice plans is based on managing the income generated by clinical faculties, billing systems are critical to the business of practice plans. The billing processes used by practice plans include single billing systems or multiple billing systems, both managed by either in-house staff or outside providers. Ninety-five percent of medical schools had a single billing system, with centralized billings and collection services for patient fees, at least at the department level. A majority of the schools, 51 percent, also had a single billing system for all physician charges. Consolidation of billing systems and physician fees proves to be the most cost-efficient, least labor-intensive method of managing a complex billing system.[35]

Managed health plans are becoming a dominant form of funding for health care benefits in the United States. Faculty practice plans are adopting the managed care structure and decision-making authority to remain competitive in the delivery of health care to patients and also to provide a patient base for FPP doctors. Managed health care plans are an integral part of cost containment efforts on the part of insurance companies and employers. These organization are increasingly appreciative of medical groups that can offer an organized, coordinated, total health care service system to their enrollees. Faculty practice plans are able to provide comprehensive services to patients in a variety of settings. This makes FPPs attractive to patient-consumers and to payees of the health care plan. As indicated in figure 3, above, almost all practice plans participate in some form of managed care.[35] More than 60 percent of practice plans are involved with a regional plan, and almost 19 percent of practice plans are involved with an HMO or an IPA. A scant 12 percent of practice plans are not involved with any managed health care. While exact data are not available, there is a tacit agreement within the managed health care industry that, the more a FPP operates as a group model, with predictable and standard fee and with governance and administrative accountability and authority, the more it is sought out as the cornerstone of their provider network.

In order to remain competitive and to be attractive to patient-consumers, FPPs are increasingly providing their services in a variety of settings: inpatient care, outpatient clinics, ambulatory care professional buildings, and satellite centers. Just as the trend toward the group model, with centralized governance and administration, is occurring as FPPs adapt to the consumer and the managed care marketplace, many FPPs are decentralizing their delivery systems not only to accommodate market demand but also to provide ambulatory care sites for medical students and resident education. Many practice plans feel it is incumbent upon them to provide services in satellite centers that are accessible by public transportation and that have generous hours of operation. These satellite centers are frequently viewed as referral sources for the schools' specialty clinics. Referrals for other health care problems are then made to the school's on-site campus location. This referral network helps ensure that referrals remain within the medical school faculty system.

As the competition for patient and health care dollars becomes more intense, faculty practice plans will need to become more creative and more aggressive in retaining and increasing their patient loads. One of the ways in which FPPs are doing this is through direct contract with employer groups. The Medical College of Wisconsin, for instance, recently negotiated a partnership health care plan with Johnson Controls, Inc., to provide patient care to its employees in four states. (In 1993, the network will expand to nine states, and eventually it will be national in scope.) By sharing a common vision, payer, patients, and providers are being organized to coordinate health care services, including preventive care, through a collaborative process for the benefit of all stakeholders. The FPPs of medical schools, appropriately structured and governed, can and should participate in health care delivery models during this time of great unrest and dissatisfaction with the rising costs and fragmentation that characterizes much of the United States's health care delivery system.

Faculty practice plans are an integral part of medical schools' financial wellbeing and future creditworthiness and are apt to be increasingly so in the future. Given that faculty practice plans will increasingly resemble the multispecialty medical group model, revenues generated by a practice plan can be independently evaluated and audited for creditworthiness. As medical schools look for new ways to finance capital expenditures and upgrade and improve medical equipment, they may find that their practice plans are a rich resource for financing these ventures.

In order to have growing and diversified income, medical schools will look increasingly toward practice plans to help them achieve their financial goals. Practice plans will need to have their own economic diversity and growth pattern. FPPs will need to evaluate the mix of their medical payees, the geographic reach of their referrals, and the breadth and growth of their medical specialties. The ability of the FPPs governance and administration to negotiate and collaborate, along with the integrity of its fee schedule, billing, and collection systems, will all be critically evaluated by credit investors. Faculty practice plans that are able to present sound financial backgrounds will keep their medical schools fiscally competitive as educational institutions, research institutions, and socially responsive clinical health care delivery systems. Research grants generate income, but they also require modern research facilities and state-of-the-art technology. Schools that are unable to remain competitive either in grants or their practice plans risk an economic cataclysm.

## References

1. Cockerham, W. *Medical Sociology.* Fourth Edition. Englewood Cliffs, N.J.: Prentice-Hall, 1989.

2. Litwin, M. Presentation on "Objective of the Faculty Practice Plan." 1991 Association of American Medical Colleges Group on Faculty Practice Professional Development Meeting, August 17, 1991.

3. D'Antuono, J. In "Group on Faculty Practice, Practice Plan Profiles." Washington, D.C.: Association of American Medical Colleges, March 1990.

4. Jolly, P., and Hudley, D. In *"AAMC Data Book Statistical Information Related to Medical Education."* Washington, D.C.: Association of American Medical Colleges, Jan. 1992.

5. D'Antuono, R. In Faculty Practice Plans: The Organization and Characteristics of Academic Medical Practice." Washington, D.C.: Association of American Medical Colleges, 1991.

*Sam J. W. Romeo, MD, MBA, FACPE, is Vice President, Clinical Practice, and Associate Dean, Clinical Affairs, Medical College of Wisconsin, Milwaukee.*

# Chapter 4

# Academic Health Centers and Their Communities: "Town and Gown"

*by Toni A. Mitchell, MD, MBA*

This chapter is divided into three segments. In order to understand the relationship of the academic health center to the community, some of the history of the development of medical education in America will be presented. Following that discussion of the growth and expansion of the medical establishment, an overview of the forces leading to the present era of competition will be presented. The third segment will be devoted to some of the approaches different academic health centers have used to meet this competition and to achieve a greater spirit of cooperation and harmony.

## Era of Growth and Development

An academic medical center is defined by the Association of Academic Health Centers as "the combination of a medical school or school of osteopathy, one or more affiliated hospitals, and at least one other health professional program (e.g., nursing or allied health)."[1] Each component of this complex organization occupies a special niche. The hospital's focus is on patients and patient care, while the academic medical center provides the governance and organizational structure. But the core of the academic health center resides in the medical school and its faculty. It is here that the melding of patient care, education, and research occurs, defining the unique character of each academic health center.[2]

The origins of medical education were much more humble. The initial practice of medicine took place primarily in patients' homes and in dispensaries. Dispensaries originated in the Eighteenth Century and were designed primarily for the poor. Funding was generally provided by the community and by philanthropists. Many physicians received their training in dispensaries while providing free care. Hospitals did not appear until the mid-Nineteenth Century and were created to provide charity bed care to the poor, especially in urban areas.[3]

Early medical education in the United States was often based on private money-making institutions, many without ties to universities. No uniform standards existed, and students' tuition fees were used to pay the lecturers.[4] However, more than 30 of the approximately 150 medical schools in existence in 1907 had full-time faculty. The primary instructional emphasis was on the basic sciences, and students were encouraged to pursue their own laboratory work and to learn by participation, not just observation. These tenets did not extend to the clinical practice, however, where most instruction remained didactic.[5] Such was the state of medical education in 1908, when Abraham Flexner undertook a study of medical education in North America under the auspices of the Carnegie Foundation for the Advancement of Teaching. Flexner's report had a far-reaching impact on how physicians were trained, because he emphasized the need for the enhanced use of clerkships for training in clinical medicine. Even more profound was his observation that teaching hospitals needed to be an integral part of universities, with full-time faculty devoted to teaching and research, not simply the private practice of medicine. And so the course was set. The Johns Hopkins Hospital and the Johns Hopkins School of Medicine, with their large endowments, clearly articulated mission, and outstanding faculty, became the standard bearers.[5] The transition of medical education from merely on-the-job training to scholarly pursuit had begun.[6]

A number of changes obviously had to take place in order to implement Flexner's recommendations. Recent advances had been made in the basic science areas because of the emphasis on the laboratory method. This led to improved conditions in hospitals, so they began offering their services to patients who could pay for them. Because doctors' fees were not included in this arrangement, some enterprising physicians (particularly surgeons) built their own hospitals.[5]

Because of continuing progress in both science and the organization of hospitals, many more services became hospital-based. In fact, some hospitals appeared to serve primarily at the behest of the private physicians who admitted patients there. But not all physicians were permitted to admit patients, so an apparent medical elite developed on the basis of admitting privileges. The medical elite included some medical school faculty members who practiced at a university hospital such as Johns Hopkins or at an affiliated hospital. This stratification based on admitting privileges and hospital fees may represent the first emergence of the "town versus gown" syndrome.[5]

At this point, medical schools had access to hospitals more often than before, but they did not control them, and severe restrictions were placed on faculty and students. Permission had to be obtained from hospitals' boards in order for instructors and their students to examine patients or participate in patient management. Generally, their participation was limited to "amphitheater lectures, ward walks, outpatient clinics, and by the turn of the century, bedside section teaching, but not by the clerkship."[5] Even a venerable institution such as Harvard was unable to persuade the board of the Massachusetts General Hospital to permit the introduction of a clerkship for medical students. Furthermore, the universities could not appoint their faculty members to their primary teaching hospital. Few universities had the resources to build their own hospitals, so clinical research and bedside teaching languished. Interestingly, the practice of obstetrics was the most advanced segment of clinical practice in the early part of this century, because most deliveries occurred at home. The resistance of hospitals to recognition of their responsibilities in medical research and education, as well as patient care, remained until World War I.[5] It is clear that, since their inception, medical schools have had a complex, and even adversarial, relationship with hospitals, physicians, and the communities in which they exist.

The academic medical center as we have come to understand it actually began in the post-World War II era, when the federal government recognized the remarkable progress that could be achieved in a short time with extensive research funding.[2] But there were patient care needs to be met along with biomedical research. The health care needs of returning veterans led to affiliations between medical schools and Veterans Administration hospitals and community hospitals, because more physicians and other health professionals were needed. There was also a perceived need to increase the academic base for the fields of nursing, pharmacy, and allied health.[1]

The impact of the federal government was significant and was exerted through four major programs: the National Institutes of Health (NIH), the Health Professions Education Acts, the Veterans Administration, and Medicare and Medicaid.[1] These initiatives greatly influenced the three major missions of the academic health center: patient care, teaching, and research.

Various health professions acts passed in the years 1951-1976 were all directed toward increasing the supply of physicians, nurses, and allied health professionals.[1] The Health Professions Educational Assistance Act of 1963 was particularly effective in increasing the numbers of health care professionals, because it provided for low-cost loans for medical, dental, and osteopathic students. Equally important, there were provisions for capital investment to improve the physical plant of hospitals and medical schools, including research facilities. Follow-up legislation in 1968 and 1971 provided financial incentives, especially in the form of capitation allowances, to increase enrollments of medical, nursing, and allied health students.[1,7] In fact, these programs "allocated $3 billion to academic medical centers between 1965 and 1980."[8]

As noted earlier, providing access to patients was the major difficulty encountered in the evolution of clinical instruction by medical schools and their faculties. As university hospitals were built and affiliations with existing community hospitals were forged, this access was achieved. Traditionally, most of these teaching hospitals provided care primarily for the poor and disadvantaged. And even in these changing times, while teaching hospitals comprise only 5.6 percent of acute care beds, they provide 47.2 percent of the care to those who are uninsured or underinsured.[9] In 1986, this represented more than $4 billion.[8] Medical centers also have traditionally served as the referral center for highly complex and difficult cases.[7] In addition, academic medical centers provide much of specialized care, because they "operate more than one-third of our nation's burn centers; supply more than half of all organ transplantation services; provide 36 percent of open-heart surgical services; and operate more than 22 percent of this country's trauma centers."[8]

The passage of legislation in 1965 creating Medicare and Medicaid altered the pattern of caring principally for charity cases. Now the elderly and poor provided much needed revenue, because of the "cost-plus" and "pass-through" provisions for academic center reimbursement. The provisions took into account the increased expense of hospitals involved in the education and training of medical students and residents. Medicare provided an adjustment for indirect medical education expenses, along with the pass-through payments for the direct medical education cost component. However, though special consideration was given to academic health centers in funding, these legislative initiatives were directed toward enhanced patient care, not research or education. Patients were provided with access to other hospitals where they would previously have been denied,[1] and this introduced an element of competition for patients.

The Department of Medicine and Surgery within the Veterans Administration was established by Congress in 1946 in order to provide high-quality care for veterans returning from World War II, as well as for those of past and future conflicts. Veterans Administration hospitals were strongly encouraged to seek affiliation with nearby local medical schools. This association was welcomed by both parties,

| Table 1. Growth of Medical School Establishment between 1960 and 1980.* | | | | | |
|---|---|---|---|---|---|
| Academic Year | No. of Schools | Total Enrollment | No. of Graduates | No. of Preclinical Faculty | No. of Full-Time Clinical Faculty |
| 1960-61 | 86 | 21,379 | 5,275 | 4,023 | 7,201 |
| 1970-71 | 101 | 30,084 | 7,081 | 8,283 | 19,256 |
| 1979-80 | 126 | 63,800 | 15,135 | 13,039 | 36,566 |
| Between 1960-61 and 1970-71 | 17% | 41% | 34% | 106% | 167% |
| Between 1970-71 and 1979-80 | 25% | 112% | 114% | 57% | 90% |
| Between 1960-61 and 1979-80 | 47% | 198% | 187% | 224% | 408% |

\* Source: Figure 3, Figure 10. In: Medical education: institutions, characteristics and programs: a background paper, Washington, DC: Association of American Medical Colleges, May 1981.

because the Veterans Administration hospitals were provided access to high-quality medical care, the prestige of affiliation with medical schools, and the opportunity to educate future physicians and research scientists. The university benefitted with expanded residency programs, increased clinical faculty, and enhanced research funding. Then, in 1976, further legislation led to the creation of five new state medical schools in association with Veterans Administration hospitals. These new medical complexes were located in areas (such as eastern Tennessee and central Ohio) where there was a perceived shortage of physicians, particularly in primary care. So, eventually, legislation governing veterans' medical affairs became consonant with the Health Professions Education Acts and Medicare and Medicaid in emphasizing patient care as the driving force. Patient care remains the underpinning for the other two missions of teaching and research, for without patients neither would be possible.[10] So, in the evolution of academic health centers, university hospitals and Veterans Administration hospitals have become the "laboratory for clinical research and the teaching of clinical medicine to students at the undergraduate and graduate levels...."[7]

Perhaps the most influential of all the federal legislation put forth, however, created the National Institutes of Health (NIH). NIH has been significant in two ways. First, it has been a major source of extramural funding for medical school faculty for several decades. In addition, NIH has trained most of this country's university investigators through its Clinical Center and its various research laboratories. Biomedical research has contributed substantially to the viability of academic health centers for many years. In fact, Colloton states that medical research funding from the federal government is approximately $4.5 billion per year, with $3.5

billion dispensed through NIH.[8] As noted by Wilson and McLaughlin, the success of this government/academia partnership has had a dramatic impact on the practice of medicine and on the development of social programs around the world.[2]

Ironically, a distinct separation of research from education in the appropriations language of the federal legislation that funds NIH has indirectly led to the present abundance of specialists at the expense of generalists, and to the paucity of funds for patient education and public policy.[2] During the era of strong research support, patient care by medical school faculties was often by referral only, creating the perception of an "ivory tower" style of medicine that resulted in almost complete isolation of academic physicians from their colleagues in the community.

Because of the strong support of the federal government in the various areas outlined, there was tremendous growth in the number of medical schools, which was followed by increases in both clinical and preclinical faculty to teach the growing number of medical students and graduate students seeking PhD degrees in medically related fields. The table on page 32 compares medical school growth in the decades 1960-1980.[1]

The contribution of the federal government to the operating budgets of most medical schools peaked at 54 percent in 1965-66, as is evident in figure 1, page 34. This drop in funding from the federal government was parallelled by a sharp rise in funds derived from practice revenue (figure 2, page 34). A watershed had been reached, and academic medical centers needed to change to meet the new challenges ahead.

## Era of Competition

Prior to the 1980s, most academic medical centers had placed minimal emphasis on the economics of delivering health care. During the Reagan Administration, many changes occurred that led to concern about the ability of academic medical centers and their university hospitals to remain viable. Pressure came from two directions: the price of delivering care and the market share of available patients. As noted by Grossman, the "price pressure" resulted from the emergence of managed care and from efforts in cost containment.[11] Both of these trends put tremendous stress on academic medical centers unable to meet the requirements of volume discounts, earlier discharges, and more outpatient evaluation. The second pressure came from increased competition for patients. As noted previously, most legislative efforts have been directed toward providing improved patient care or increased access, not subsidization of medical education or academic health centers.

Many of the changes that were contemplated (a great number of which were implemented) forced academic health centers into direct competition with the remainder of the medical communities in which they were located, and "town versus gown" controversy erupted to varying degrees in nearly every academic medical center. As noted previously, university hospitals provide care to a disproportionate share of the indigent population, and the medical community at large has considered this to be the rightful role of the teaching hospital. But with decreasing sources of funding for this free care, teaching hospitals have begun to develop strategies to attract paying patients. This change in the traditional role of the teaching hospital has created conflict between community physicians and hospitals and the university hospital. Many teaching hospitals have attempted to encourage nonteaching hospitals, especially not-for-profit institutions, to shoulder more of the load of charity care. The federal government has supported this initiative with OBRA and COBRA legislation that prevents hospitals' emergency departments from refusing care to patients who present requesting medical treatment.

Still, academic health centers have created their own major competition by training a large cadre of highly trained specialists who can provide most of the care previously reserved for academic institutions.[9] Many faculty members are now

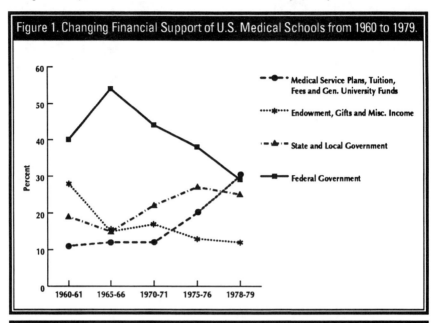

Figure 1. Changing Financial Support of U.S. Medical Schools from 1960 to 1979.

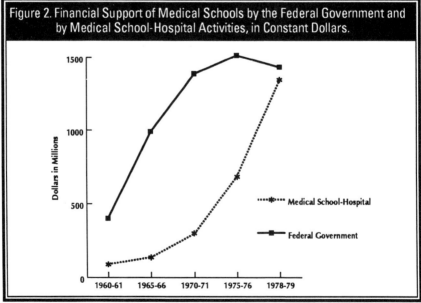

Figure 2. Financial Support of Medical Schools by the Federal Government and by Medical School-Hospital Activities, in Constant Dollars.

in direct competition with their former trainees who are practicing at community hospitals that are better equipped to respond rapidly to changing patient demands and market forces.

Another major problem area has been the lack of communication between university-based physicians and their community counterparts. As Carey notes, faculty members are often not as communicative as their counterparts with referring physicians.[7] And academic physicians often are isolated by their own choice when they do not join the county medical society and other state or regional medical groups where relationships with referring physicians could be developed. This lack of communication has often led to the continuing stereotype of the supercilious academic physician on the one hand, and the LMD (local medical doctor) or "boondocs" on the other.

Members of faculty practice plans and the administrators of academic medical centers have failed to communicate their changing circumstances and evolving needs to other physicians. Most nonuniversity physicians were trained in academic medical centers, and remember them as they were in previous years. Most of them never anticipated that they would be confronted by competition from university physicians during the course of their practice. Neither did they anticipate the marked increase in regulation, quality assurance, managed care, and prospective payment. But physicians generally change attitudes and practices when given the necessary information; the university community must reach out to its nonuniversity colleagues in increased dialogue to permit this understanding to develop.

Finally, the reward systems under which the two groups operate have been very different. For the community physician, the rewards have come through developing relationships with patients and other physicians. University physicians have generally looked to the intellectual challenge of research and the education of the next generation of physicians, which usually has led to job security through the promotion and tenure process. Although both groups desire to promote the best medical care possible for patients, academic physicians have been perceived as strong in the "science" of medicine, and community physicians better in the "art" of medicine.

## Era of Solutions and Cooperation
In the mid-1980s, Johns Hopkins Hospital recognized that the practice environment for academic institutions was about to be thrown into turmoil. So it developed and implemented a plan that included both vertical and horizontal integration in order to meet the hospital's need to maintain a strong financial footing and the medical school's need for an expanded patient base, especially in ambulatory care.[12] Vertical integration was achieved through acquisitions that enabled Johns Hopkins to provide both acute and chronic care through its hospital system and home health care, as well as primary care and specialty care through its clinics, health maintenance organization, and preferred provider network. Horizontal integration was accomplished through the acquisition of other hospitals.

A holding company, the Johns Hopkins Health System, was established to oversee the acquisition and operations of the various insurance products, Francis Scott Key Medical Center (previously Baltimore City Hospitals), North Charles General Hospital and the Wyman Park Health System (previously a United States Public Health Service facility), a home health agency, and a chronic care facility. These changes did not occur without strain between the hospital and the medical school, but both were dedicated to preserving the principles of excellent patient care leading to world class research and medical education.[13] The Johns Hopkins approach was to totally integrate itself into the health care delivery system at all levels. As a result, a large number of community physicians were brought under Johns Hopkins' institutional umbrella with the acquisition of the health maintenance organization and other hospitals.

Other institutions have used differing approaches. The University of Southern California (USC) has attempted to make its facilities "user friendly" and its faculty approachable. It has developed the Physician Access and Communication Exchange (PACE), which provides 24-hour-a-day availability of consultants to answer questions and offer clinical information/advice to community physicians regarding difficult patients. A similar system (MIST) has been in place at the University of Alabama in Birmingham (UAB) for a number of years. This give-and-take has improved communications between community physicians and the university faculty and increased referrals to the University Hospital faculty at both USC and UAB.[14]

Although the medical staff of the University of Southern California's University Hospital is restricted to members of the medical school faculty practice plan, some exceptions are made for clinical faculty. Private patients are admitted to this facility, and outpatient services are also available. USC has been able to make this process feasible by encouraging referral of complex cases from community physicians, thereby avoiding direct competition for primary care patients. University faculty members are expected to see these referral patients themselves, and the patients are returned to the original referring physician after the evaluation. The expectation is that the communication between the university faculty and the referring community physician will be gracious, prompt, and thorough.

Because University Hospital is relatively new, the hospital and the medical school have an active campaign to educate local physicians and other health care facilities about its unique features and elect not to go straight to the public. The chairs of the clinical departments are dedicated to effective communication with community physicians who refer patients. If a private patient or the private patient's physician wants to reach attending physician from the USC faculty, the faculty member is available and there is no "screening out" process. The chairs also recognize the need to provide efficient, high-quality medical care to patients.

A unique aspect of the relationship between the university faculty and community physicians at USC is an organization named Salerni Collegium, which was founded by the private physicians. The group comprises university and private physicians who are dedicated to the financial support of the medical school; each member pays annual dues. In addition to the financial aspect, the most valuable feature may be the simple opportunity for the physicians to network with one another. Furthermore, the university invites prominent local community physicians to present grand rounds and conduct roundtable discussions on different topics of interest to both groups.[14]

The Hillsborough County Medical Association (of the Florida Medical Association) has established a Liaison Committee to help recruit more members from the University of South Florida College of Medicine faculty. If successful, this increased contact between the large local medical community and the university faculty should lead to improved communication and a better understanding of the stresses presently being placed on all physicians. Ideally, this outreach program will provide a forum for developing trust and respect for the work that each individual performs.

Most academic health centers have some voluntary clinical faculty members, but the composition of this faculty and the expectations of its members' performance vary widely. Barondess has suggested that clinical faculty can fill a number of roles in academia, including clinical teaching, instruction in physical diagnosis, attending clinical rounds on inpatient services, and supervision of outpatient ambulatory clinics. He notes that voluntary and full-time faculty are alike in many ways, particularly in their commitment to excellence.[15] Appropriate inclusion of clinical faculty members could be a boon to university centers as an added resource, but their presence also provides the ideal environment for developing university/community ties and for exposing medical students to the complexities of the day-to-day practice of medicine.

Reward systems within the university appear to have changed little over the past 50 years, and discussions with present leaders in academic health centers seem to confirm that research productivity and publications in scholarly journals represent the major portion of tenure and promotion decisions.[15,16] This seems, at least in part, to be due to the ease of measurement of this output compared with excellence in teaching, patient care, or service to the institution and community. But change is inevitable, driven by the very excellence that has prevailed over the past years. It is difficult for a physician to be a part-time researcher and a part-time clinician. Physicians are rapidly being overtaken by PhD scientists who pursue their laboratory investigations full-time. This transition is demonstrated by the 11 percent increase in research grants awarded to PhD scientists by NIH between 1970 and 1987.[10]

Other pressures for change in the reward system arise from the increased need to fund other endeavors of the academic institution from patient care revenue. Recognition of the need to separate the physician-scientist and clinician-scholar led the Department of Internal Medicine at the University of Michigan to create two faculty development tracks. Clearly, physician-scientists need large amounts of protected time for research in order to be able to compete successfully for research funds. However, this tenure-earning track entails a specific commitment of time to medical education as well. A parallel tenure-earning track was developed for the clinician-scholar, whose time is divided among medical education, provision of clinical services, and some research activities. Both tracks were recognized as vital to the success of the department, and provisions were made for transfer between the two tracks if criteria were met and the individual desired such a transfer. Since the inception of this system in 1977, two nontenure tracks have also been established. Full-time clinical track physicians devote virtually all of their time to patient care activities, primarily at off-site clinics. A full-time research track, primarily for nonphysician scientists, was developed. Additionally, emeritus and leadership tracks were identified for senior faculty. The keys to success of this arrangement appear to have been the flexibility to adapt to a changing environment, clear delineation of the requirements for each track, and emphasis on the equal importance of all tracks to the success of the Department and College as a whole.[17]

Thus, in many instances, the reward systems of the nonuniversity community physician are now being integrated into the promotion and tenure decisions of major academic institutions. Perhaps this alignment will result in better understanding of the role of each, rather than increased strife due to the competitive nature of this change.

Over the past 50 years, government largess has permitted rapid growth of the medical establishment, and the academic health center has been a centerpiece of that development. Society has granted academic institutions great autonomy and rewarded them with substantial financial support. In return, society has received the best that organized medicine has to offer: well-trained physicians to care for their health needs; major advances in scientific and technical knowledge to extend life expectancy and enhance the quality of life; and excellent patient care, regardless of the ability to pay, as well as pioneering efforts in fields not imagined 50 years ago, such as organ transplantation.[8]

Society's expectation of medicine, particularly the academic medical center, is changing. As a result, the relationship of the academic medical center with the community at large is being redefined, and it is a painful process. While we are expected to continue to care for the nearly 37 million people in the United States without insurance, we are expected to do so with decreasing government support and without shifting costs to those who do pay. Additionally, medical schools are expected to provide top-quality graduates who will increasingly represent minorities and women, even though private philanthropy and scholarships are unavailable to overcome the high costs and resultant debt incurred in obtaining a medical education. Furthermore, university hospitals are still expected to remain on the "cutting edge" of patient care and technology, although no one wants to pay the higher prices this inevitably entails.[8]

We can, and must, meet these challenges from our communities. Academic medical centers must be vigilant, ensuring that medical education does not revert to the pre-Flexner days, when the private practice of medicine consumed all the physician's time and effort, thereby losing its necessary grounding in scholarly pursuits. And we must not relegate our students to the status of observers only, as they were in the days before clerkships.

Much of medicine's future success will require significant, visible community involvement to reestablish the trust many physicians, hospitals, and medical schools have lost in this age of competition and apparent selfishness. Support of the community, local and beyond, should take many forms. Academic health centers need to continue to provide care for the needy and disenfranchised of the community. But members of the academic community need to be visible patient advocates as well. Pediatricians can be involved with children's advocacy groups and emergency physicians and trauma surgeons with trauma legislation. Major academic centers have been vocal advocates of better housing for the poor and improved job opportunities.

Teaching hospitals have always provided much more to the community than medical care. They have also met many of the social needs of their patients. Social workers help patients, many of them non-English speaking, negotiate the maze of hospitals, clinics, public health facilities, and state health agencies in order to get the care that they need.

Grossman comments that, "Community service is our bond with the past and our hope for the future. And I for one have no doubt that our future will be bright. Ralph Waldo Emerson once wrote of his own era, 'This time, like all times, is a very good one, if we but know what to do with it.'"[11]

# References

1.  Ebert, R., and Brown, S. "Academic Health Centers." *New England Journal of Medicine.* 308(20):1200-8, May 19, 1983.

2.  Wilson, M., and McLaughlin, C. "Managing a National Resource: Demands on Academic Medicine." In *Leadership and Management in Academic Medicine.* San Francisco, Calif.: Jossey-Bass Publishers, 1984, pp. 3-38.

3.  Marchant, D. "Academia—An Endangered Species." *American Journal of Obstetrics and Gynecology.* 156(1):185-92, Jan. 1987.

4.  Lovell, R. "The University Medical Presence in Hospitals Seventy Years After Flexner and a Look Ahead." *Australian and New Zealand Journal of Medicine* 13(2):187-94, April 1983.

5.  Ludmerer, K. "The Plight of Clinical Teaching in America." *Bulletin of the History of Medicine* 57(2):218-29, Summer 1983.

6.  DiBiaggio, J. "A 20-Year Forecast for Academic Medical Centers." *New England Journal of Medicine* 304(4):228-30, Jan. 21, 1981.

7.  Carey, L. "Presidential Address: The Academic Medical Center—Dynasty or Dinosaur?" *Surgery* 102(4):555-60, Oct. 1987.

8.  Colloton, J. "Academic Medicine's Changing Covenant with Society." *Academic Medicine* 64(2):55-60, Feb. 1989.

9.  Rogers, D., and Blendon, R. "The Academic Medical Center Today." *Annals of Internal Medicine* 100(5):751-4, May 1984.

10. Sadeghi-Nejad, A., and Marquardt, M. "Academic Physicians: Today's Dinosaurs?" *American Journal of Medicine* 90(3):371-3, March 1991.

11. Grossman, J. "Community Commitment, Competition, and the Future of Academic Medical Centers." *Inquiry* 23(3):245-52, Fall 1986.

12. Heyssel, R. "Changing Environment and the Academic Medical Center: The Johns Hopkins Hospital." *Academic Medicine* 64(1):7-11, Jan. 1989.

13. Ross, R., and Johns, M. "Changing Environment and the Academic Medical Center: The Johns Hopkins School of Medicine." *Academic Medicine* 64(1):1-6, Jan. 1989.

14. Spears, R. Personal communication, Nov. 1991.

15. Barondess, J. "Voluntary Clinical Faculty. The Hope of the Future?" *Archives of Internal Medicine* 143(2):338-40, Feb. 1983.

16. Hartfield, J. Personal communication, Nov. 1991.

17. Kelley, W., and Stross, J. "Faculty Tracks and Academic Success." *Annals of Internal Medicine* 116(8):654-9, April 15, 1992.

# Further Reading

Cadman, E. "Who Will Determine the Future of Academic Medicine?" *Clinical Research* 34(3):415-20, Sept. 1986.

Cooper, J. "What Is Immediate Past Is Prologue—Unfortunately." *Journal of Medical Education* 61(2):112-8, Feb. 1986.

Daniels, R. "The Future of the Academic Health Science Center." *Ohio State Medical Journal* 78(3):167, March 1982.

Ebert, R., and Ginzberg, E. "The Reform of Medical Education." *Health Affairs* 7(2,Supplement):5-38, 1988.

Foreman, S. "Graduate Medical Education: Focus for Change." *Academic Medicine* 65(2):77-84, Feb. 1990.

Petersdorf, R., and Wilson, M. "The Four Horsemen of the Apocalypse. Study of Academic Medical Center Governance." *JAMA* 247(8):1153-61, Feb. 26, 1982.

Petersdorf, R. "Three Easy Pieces." *Academic Medicine* 65(2):73-7, Feb. 1990.

Rogers, D. "On Preparing Academic Health Centers for the Very Different 1980s." *Journal of Medical Education* 55(1):1-12, Jan. 1980.

Swales, J. "What Has Happened to Academic Medicine?" *Lancet* 1(8491):1194-6, May 24, 1986.

Turner, B. "Future Role of Academic Medical Centers." *Health Care Management Review* 14(2):73-7, Spring 1989.

Tyson, K., and Merrill, J. "Health Care Institutions: Survival in a Changing Environment." *Journal of Medical Education* 59(10):773-82, Oct. 1984.

*Toni A. Mitchell, MD, MBA, is Medical Director, Adult Emergency Care Center, Tampa General Hospital, Tampa, Florida. She is also Clinical Assistant Professor of Medicine, University of South Florida, Tampa. She serves as Vice Chair of the ACPE Forum for Women in Medicine and Management and is a member of the Review Panel of the ACPE Society on Academic Health Centers. Dr. Mitchell extends her heartfelt thanks to James Hartfield, MD, FACPE, Associate Vice President of Medical Affairs, University of South Florida Health Sciences Center, Tampa; Robert Spears, MD, FACPE, Associate Dean, Clinical Affairs, University of Southern California School of Medicine, Los Angeles; and Thomas McKell, MD, Vice President and Medical Director, Tampa General Hospital, Tampa, Florida, for their contributions to this chapter.*

# Chapter 5

# Strategic Planning and External Markets

*by Marjorie P. Wilson, MD, FACPE,
and Curtis P. McLaughlin, DBA*

**S**trategic planning is a management function and a process, not a product. It involves identifying the critical objectives that define institutional purpose and shape the organizational direction of the academic medical center.[1] The process must be a dynamic, visionary, continuous one based on critical objectives and available opportunities. Strategic planning is the process that answers major policy and resource questions relative to the future directions and principal opportunities of the organization.

The essential elements for the successful use of strategic planning in academic medical centers appear to include:

■ Accurate knowledge of the internal and external environment and of the viewpoints of its many relevant internal and external constituencies.

■ Top leadership's involvement as well as that of many of the key implementers in the planning process.

■ Commitment to a broad, but focused, set of objectives, usually articulated as a defined mission based on the competencies and values of the organization.

■ A vision of what the institution is and could become.

■ A process aimed at decision making and implementation.

■ A process for making sure that internal and external communities are informed of the vision and the mission as it evolves.

■ Realism in resources, time, and feasibility.

■ Process improvement as an intended outcome—both the institution's processes of delivery of its services and the planning process itself.

■ Change as an anticipated result—changes in priorities, policies, activities, and power relationships.

Another key element of successful strategic planning is management of any unrealistic expectations: for example, that planning can control the environment. Faculty and administration must try to influence external events and decisions, but this process can prove very destructive, should people fantasize that strategic planning would permit them to act as free agents in the future. An academic medical center is always in flux. There are never-ending sets of crises, problems, and opportunities: conflicts to resolve; people, money, and space to acquire and allocate; and key people coming and leaving. It is a "process world," where "every solution to a problem becomes a problem of its own."[2]

Among the expectations to be managed are those held by the external world. This introduces the concept of "marketing." Drucker summarizes these key relationships as follows:

"We hear a great deal these days about leadership, and it's high time we did. But, actually, mission comes first. Non-profit institutions exist for the sake of their mission. They exist to make a difference in society and the life of the individual. They exist for the sake of their mission, and this must never be forgotten.

"...Despite its importance, however, many nonprofits tend to slight strategy....too many non-profit managers confuse strategy with a selling effort. Strategy ends with selling efforts. It begins with knowing the market—who the customer is, who the customer should be, who the customer might be. The whole point of strategy is not to look at recipients as people who receive bounty, to whom the non-profit does good. They are customers who have to be satisfied. The non-profit institution needs a marketing strategy that integrates the customer and the mission.

"...An effective non-profit institution also needs strategies to improve all the time and to innovate. The two overlap.

"...And then the non-profit institution needs a strategy to build its donor base. It needs to develop a donor constituency.

"...All three of these strategies begin with research, research and more research."[3]

Gallagher and Weinberg note that:

"...the most significant difference between business and nonprofits is the one that actually generates all the complications. Nonprofits have more complex missions than do businesses. The marketing challenges that arise as a result can almost all be dealt with effectively by appealing to the organizational mission. Consequently, the importance of a well thought-out, clearly articulated, and deeply understood mission cannot be overstated. Ultimately, that is the source of success for nonprofits."[4]

## Definitions

### What Is an Academic Medical Center?

Before going further, we should define the model we will use to analyze the strategic planning process. The academic medical center is an organizational complex made up of a medical school; usually one but sometimes several teaching hospitals; and additional semiautonomous research institutes and centers, clinics, and ambulatory care facilities. It may also include extended care facilities and a variety of other not-for-profit or even some for-profit enterprises. Many academic medical centers (or academic health centers) have other health professions schools as well. The majority of academic medical centers are university-based, although some of the nonacademic facilities may not be university-owned. The medical school invariably is one of the most influential institutions in the conglomerate and its faculty carries out its mission of education, research, and patient care in the facilities just mentioned.

The complexity of these arrangements and the diffusion of power that accompanies it are daunting. The manager who initiates and leads the strategic planning process may be the dean of the medical school, a vice president or president at the center level, or a director of the major teaching hospital. In this chapter, we focus on the academic medical center and describe activities in that context, but the principles involved in strategic planning, which we believe apply in any setting and at multiple levels of an organization, are seen as a critical management function.

## Strategy

Strategy involves identification, definition, and marshalling of the means to achieve the objectives of the organization. Strategy, therefore, must support all the major goals of the organization, not just those that support the ends of the people who work there.[5] Vancil[6] defines strategy as follows: "The strategy of an organization or of *a subunit of a larger organization* is a conceptualization, *expressed or implied by the organization's leader*, of (1) the long-term objectives or purpose of the organization, (2) the broad constraints and policies, *either self-imposed by the leader or accepted by him or her from superiors*, that *currently* restrict the organization's abilities, and (3) the *current* set of plans and near-term goals that have been adopted in the expectation of contributing to the achievement of the organization's objectives." The italics are Vancil's, designed to emphasize that strategy is necessary at all organizational levels and that strategy is not handed down permanently carved in stone.

There are two operational tests of a strategic plan. First, it must enable the organization to say no when it should. Second, it must provide a sense of cohesion. The many publics of the academic medical center place many conflicting demands and opportunities before it. Management must have a rationale for grasping some and letting others go by. The strategic plan should provide the spotter's chart for good and bad opportunities, as well as the reasons for justifying any refusals.

"The primary source of cohesiveness in an organization is strategy. To be effective it must be more than just a ringing statement of purpose and objectives....(It) should help mold an organization together by developing among the members of the management team both a shared belief in the efficacy of major action programs and a shared commitment to execute those programs effectively."[6] Cohesion is especially important in an academic medical center, where many objectives are determined environmentally and professionally, rather than organizationally. It takes leadership to accomplish this, leadership capable of managing and motivating a planning process, communicating its outcomes, and focusing people's attention toward implementation.

## Planning and Control

Planning and control are the processes of deciding what to do (planning) and ensuring that the desired results are achieved (control). They are two aspects of a continuous and iterative process. There is little use planning unless one is prepared to implement that plan and little use implementing unless the objectives are clear and worthwhile.

Planning and control occur at all levels of the organization. The research scientist must plan a series of experiments and control them. A division chief needs a scheme (plan) to raise money to pay salaries and replace equipment. A faculty needs to foresee what activities it will value highly (plan) and, by manipulating appointments and rewards (control), ensure that the right people to attain those objectives are recruited and retained. Trustees must make decisions about the sorts of activities that should be supported to meet the needs of the institution's constituencies.[5]

Anthony[7] defined three subfunctions of planning and control as:

■ Strategic planning—the process of deciding on objectives for an organization or changes in the objectives; on the resources that will be used to attain the objectives; and on the policies that govern the acquisition, use, and disposition of the resources.

■ Management control—he process by which managers ensure that the necessary resources are acquired and used effectively and efficiently in accomplishing the organization's objectives.

■ Operational control—the process of ensuring that individual tasks are carried out efficiently and effectively.

## Incrementalism, Crisis Management, and Strategic Management of Crises

In the absence of strategic planning, organizations manage by making pragmatic, ad hoc decisions—that is, by incrementalism. The rate of change in academic medical centers is so great that the most natural mode of decision making is crisis management, reacting when unanticipated situations demand immediate attention. Crises will happen in an academic medical center, and managing crises is a constructive management skill. Medicine involves real people with real crises. There are, however, many unnecessary crises that come about whenever management is not focused, does not plan, and does not have the right control mechanisms in place to match its strategic plans.

"The strength of the institution is manifest in its ability to respond flexibly to unanticipated problems and in its ability to turn a problem into an opportunity. Good strategic planning can provide the basis for more effective problem-solving by providing a framework for anticipating problems and by generating alternative solutions to issues that may lend themselves to resolution of unexpected obstacles."[8]

### Long-Range Planning and Strategic Planning

Many people use the terms "long-range planning" and "strategic planning" interchangeably and miss the essential difference between the two. When thinking about strategy, one tends to use a longer time perspective than for managerial and operational decisions, but the result is not necessarily a five- or ten-year plan, especially in the rapidly changing environment of an academic medical center. The planning horizon for a strategy may be short or long, depending on the situation. Long-range plans do not necessarily address strategic issues. Long-range planning is often formal, paper-driven, and associated with nonstrategic decisions, such as space management or facilities planning, that should be the result of strategic decision-making.

Mintzberg[9] says that "strategy formulation does not turn out to be the regular, continuous, systematic process depicted in so much of the planning literature. It is most often an irregular discontinuous process proceeding in fits and starts. There are periods of stability in strategy development, but there are also periods of flux, of groping, of piecemeal change, and of global change. To my mind, a 'strategy' represents the mediating force between the dynamic environment and a stable operating system. Strategy is the organization's 'conception' of how to deal with its environment for a while."

Mintzberg notes that a creative strategy is often a "gestalt strategy," someone's synthesis of how an organization fits into its environment. It is also called vision. Typically, a gestalt strategy is not a linear, step-by-step process; it is the product of someone's intuition. As such, it is very hard to communicate, leading to a dilemma of delegation. Especially when a strategy is unusually creative, lack of understanding of this intuition by the implementers may make them unwilling or even unable to proceed.

Long-range planning, on the other hand, does not necessarily address strategy. Often it produces a formal, rational, and static set of documents, usually descriptive and with appropriate numbers that project out into the future, three to five years or so, the management decisions already made. Such planning documents can be updated annually and still represent no change in direction unless a new set of strategic decisions are made.

### Communicating the Strategy
Communicating the strategy is a continuous task of leadership. In the ambiguous or complicated situations so common in academic medical centers, people delay to find out what the leadership thinks before taking any action. Strategies will not be implemented effectively unless institutional leadership is successful in (1) articulating the strategy clearly and (2) communicating the strategy, essentially their vision, throughout the organization.

## Scanning the Environment
An institution operates in a vacuum unless its leaders are constantly observing what is happening in the external environment. Much of the planning in an academic medical center occurs in response to external pressures, regulations, and decisions. Providing leadership requires scanning the environment and monitoring key areas outside medical center control and using this information to reformulate objectives, modify plans, and focus communications.

### Choosing the Vision
Medicine is at a major crossroads in 1992. Health care has become a pivotal political issue. More and more individuals from all political parties forecast major changes in the structure of medical care before the turn of the century. With any changes will come new roles, new risks, new opportunities for academic medical centers. Leadership will have to generate and articulate new visions to guide these institutions.

How that vision will be specifically defined we do not know, but we agree in general with the historical and sociological analysis of Rosemary Stevens[10] that the basic conflict in American medicine is between two models. The first is:

"...a model of hospitals as a supply-driven, technological system analogous to an electrification system or a system for producing military aircraft. Hospitals produce surgery, procedures, x-rays, expertise, even babies....the other is a model of hospitals as community services, with lingering religious, humanitarian, and egalitarian goals, more analogous to a system of schools.

"...Older notions of scientific medicine on which the profession and hospitals have been based—grounded in assumptions about infectious disease and surgery at the turn of the century—are no longer adequate. Resolving present problems of uncertainty (and low morale) in the American medical profession requires nothing less than the development of a revised body of theory, targeted to chronic disease, care as well as cure, and a restatement of the meaning of professionalism.

"If medicine takes the road of technological reductionism, hospitals are likely to develop as factories of human repair. If medicine becomes more socially, psychologically, and behaviorally oriented, hospitals will find it easier to grow in these directions. Doctor-hospital relations pose problems for the immediate future. There is a sense among both doctors and hospital managers that they are antagonists engaged in a power struggle, which managers expect to win. However, as in the past, the strongest institutions promise to be those where mutual accommodations are negotiated."

Jeanne M. Liedtka, in her paper on "Formulating Hospital Strategy: Moving Beyond a Market Mentality," suggests that a strategic planning process incorporating an exclusively market-driven focus is inappropriate, even dangerous, for hospitals. Instead, she argues for recognition of the "personal and professional values of the key implementers of any strategic choice and acknowledges a set of societal responsibilities related to them."[11]

As we listen to those with a historical perspective, we note attention being focused on the social responsibility of academic medicine. Not since the Sixties have we heard as much talk of the social contract of the medical school with the community, but it can be a welcome change to undertake an agenda that legitimizes the values of the profession and permits a respite from the pure business mentality imposed by the hegemony of the managed care systems of the Eighties. A decade ago, Lewis and Sheps advocated a mission in addition to research, education, and patient care—community service.[12] A first step in developing a strategy is for academic medicine to determine, in consultation with its publics, its role(s) in society.

This is not to say our teaching hospitals, clinics, medical schools and their departments, and research programs need not be managed with efficiency and effectiveness. They must be, and they cannot be excused for excesses and carelessness. But in choosing the vision for the last decade of this century, academic medicine is being asked to reconstruct its social contract with the community that supports it in its educational, research, and patient care programs.[10,13-15] This is an uncommon opportunity that should be grasped.

## Developing a Planning Process

Although there are many ways to take on the roles of leadership, eventually someone must:

■ Initiate the planning process and be responsible for its implementation.

■ Commit adequate resources (people and money) to support the process.

■ Manage the conflicts that undoubtedly will follow any proposed changes.

■ Develop or procure individual and group process skills to formulate strategy and doable goals.

■ Gain the cooperation of neutral or negatively disposed participants and perhaps be prepared to replace or at least isolate the uncooperative ones.

■ See that the strategy is referred to repeatedly as the context for most, if not all, major decisions.

■ Renew the process if it lapses or if a new iteration seems due.

Planning is an integral part of the management process, not an "add-on." If it is taken seriously, its results will be implemented through hundreds of day-to-day decisions. Managers who disparage planning do not understand their functional responsibility.

### Managing Conflicts

Debating objectives and preparing plans creates conflicts. So does the process of allocating resources. It is up to managers to have the "will to manage," to deal with the conflicts produced, to manage them rather than avoid them.[16] This involves being willing to exhibit by word, and more especially by behavior, the way people are expected to treat problems and each other. It implies a number of values and behaviors that go beyond bureaucratic functioning. Bower further articulated the will to manage as including (1) being alert to the external forces at work on the organization; (2) being decisive, taking risks to avoid delay, accompanied by a willingness to admit and correct mistakes; (3) seizing and exploiting opportunity, but going beyond pragmatism, staying within the gestalt of where the organization is heading; and (4) seeking out and facing up to problems, including difficult people decisions, that implies being fair and not ruthless, but not suffering fools or poor performance gladly.

Conflict is an existential problem in any adapting, changing, healthy organization. Beckhard and Harris[17] argue that one sign of a healthy organization is high situational conflict, but low interpersonal conflict. The situational conflict comes from high standards and a high activity level. One way that effective managers keep interpersonal conflict down is by interpreting situational conflicts to staff. Leaders must continually interpret environmental forces and internal activities in a way that allows individual employees to face up to the nature of their situations and to the gains and losses at stake. Leaders must confront individuals taking events personally and persuade them not to develop cliques nor become enemies over situational outcomes. This can be a tall order in a medical environment, where long training periods and high professional identification often lead to poorly developed differentiation between one's professional and personal personae.

### Managers Conditioned by Medical Experience

Effective decision making is a skill demanded of both physicians and administrators, but the functional differences between patient care management and institutional management should be clearly understood. Successful physicians have learned to respond to their challenges like fine racehorses. Used to working in short bursts, with direct, hands-on control of situations, they are doers. In the patient care setting, the physician is personally responsible for or has control over many, if not all, aspects of the decision-making process. The physician is viewed as the legitimate person to determine the course of treatment and command the resources necessary to implement it. Society has conferred that responsibility and authority on the basis of unique expertise. However, administrative decision making in professional organizations, such as academic medical centers, depends or relies on norms of shared stewardship. Before action is taken, some level of agreement has to be reached about the definition of the problem, the alternatives to be considered, and the resources to be used. Society's conferring of authority and responsibility to physicians does not extend into the administrative sphere. The public understands its limited ability to evaluate diagnostic and therapeutic choices, but it feels qualified to judge administrative performance. It does so, albeit imperfectly, at the polls each year.

Administrative decision making, therefore, is often frustrating and diffuse in an academic medical center, requiring the involvement of multiple and often competing advocates at many levels. The process tends to be a slow one based on negotiation, education, and compromise, often frustrating to those who are trained to deal with a presented problem in a short time and then move on to the next problem.

### Developing the Individual and Group Planning Process

Even when there is adequate time to devote to strategic planning, it is not a solitary process. Effective implementation depends on the implementers' having participated in the planning process enough to feel they own it, to want to make it work, to choose to persuade others to make it work. An implementation-oriented planning process, therefore, requires development of a governance-related group process, with an explicit faculty role. Given the diffuseness of power in the academic medical center and the frailty of trust in its leadership, the dean, chair, or vice president cannot lead solely by giving orders or issuing rewards and punishments.

It is the leader's responsibility to set and communicate the objectives of the organization (which will create conflict), to allocate its resources (which will again create conflict), and then to manage that conflict by personal example, by structure, intervention, and particularly by demonstrating understanding of the values and professionalism of the principal players, i.e. those who do the teaching, do the research and bring in its support, and, last but not least, do the patient care and bring a significant amount of monetary support to the hospitals and the medical school. The leader must use all the resources he or she can command, including:

■ Personal resources—intelligence, honor, verbal skill, and charm.

■ Situational resources—knowledge, contacts, timing, opportunity, aided especially by:

- Knowledge of the institution and the climate within which it operates.

- Technical expertise.

- Ability to define clearly issues and managerial tasks.
- Clear articulation of responsibilities and authorities.

■ Enabling resources—especially staff.

Having planning resources gives the leader choices as to which roles to play directly in the planning process and which to delegate, choices that also depend on the issues, the staff available, and the leader's managerial style. Many strategic planning efforts have gone awry because planning for planning has been inadequate.

There are many options available for planning, including:

■ A planning staff.

■ The senior manager as planner.

■ Standing committee(s).

■ Ad hoc task forces.

■ Combinations of the above.

The first approach that often comes to mind is the use of a specialized planning staff. Yet that alternative all too often leads to lots of paper and little organizational change if it does not involve the implementers. The better approach is for the vice president or dean or chair to take on the role of planner-in-chief and then delegate the many tasks involved to committees and to staff personnel. Many organizations do poorly with the structure and function of staff participation, especially committees. When planning experts such as Vancil and Lorange[6] speak of getting the right people together at the right time, often they are referring to the intricacies of managing the governance and the committee-based processes. Delbecq and Gill,[18] writing of community-based physicians, noted that fairness for them was embodied in a process that (1) took little of their personal time, but in which they were represented; (2) took place in the open; and (3) resulted in clear decision rules. Those are good criteria for the planning process as well.

Shortell[19] has analyzed the structural and governance issues in depth and has suggested a "parallel organization" for a hospital's governance. Because of the complexity and cross-cutting nature of organizational issues, he suggests a matching complex of committees involving medical staff to help govern and motivate the institution. The planning process is one component of the approach that he suggests.

On a more pragmatic basis, Cunliff and Smith[20] suggest that a high level of staff involvement in a hospital is necessary to gain the support of physicians and to guard against fits and starts in planning when top management turns over.

### Managing Committees

Managing committees is like managing research, which rests on getting the right people in the first place, the people who are passionately interested in accomplishing the same ends that you are. Then you can give them abundant autonomy. One problem with committees is that most are given too many roles to handle simultaneously within one group: (1) representation of interests and power blocs, (2) information gathering, (3) analytical and problem-solving assignments, (4) influencing opinion and commitment among the implementers, and (5) influencing opinion and commitment among the organizational hierarchy.

The 7 to 12 persons who make up the maximum-sized working committee cannot possibly wear all these hats at once and still function effectively. The complex objectives and constituencies in an academic medical center often require the involvement of different people from different levels of the organization during different phases of the process. The figure below illustrates one arrangement that a dean might use for planning. It is only one of many alternatives and is not presented as an ideal. Each situation will be different and have its own possibilities.

In the situation in the figure, the dean has chosen at the first stage to be planner-in-chief and the catalyst who stimulates the process. He or she appoints an ad hoc committee to start the process and to define the problems of the institution. Committee members are likely to be selected on the basis of three criteria: (1) as representatives of interests (e.g. tenured vs. nontenured faculty), (2) for influence as opinion leaders among the faculty, and (3) for adaptability to the process of strategic planning. The committee develops the agenda with input from the dean

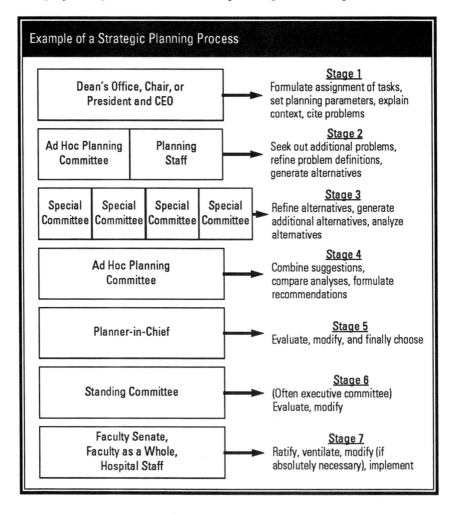

and support from the planning staff of the dean's office. Such a committee is likely to represent a diagonal slice of the organization, cutting across departments and ranks.[21] Still its members find that they do not have access to all much-needed information or to all the relevant implementers. So they develop a series of special ad hoc committees focused on specific issues, made up of the people who are closest to the appropriate information and who will lead the implementation. These committees generate more information and more detailed alternatives, again working hand-in-hand with planning staff members, who serve as analysts and, in some limited cases, as advisers. Careful attention must be given to making sure that standing committees, such as the curriculum committee, are not bypassed by these committees.

Once special and standing committees have developed suggestions, they need to check with the chief executive to make sure that they are not off base. Acting as chief evaluator and strategist, the leader can judge whether or not the committees are on an acceptable tack and suggest additional factors, issues, or alternatives to be considered at this point. Once the committees and the leader are satisfied, the results can be presented to the formal hierarchy—the chairs and division chiefs.

The formal hierarchy cannot do the planning alone, because its members are so involved in representing and protecting their areas of interest that they will have trouble with the problem-solving and analytical phases .of the planning process. Some will be on specific committees in their roles as experts, information sources, or opinion leaders, but a hierarchical planning committee, made up of persons of top rank, is unlikely to come up with innovative planning, especially in a climate of scarce resources. A number of centers have already found that, in a time of declining resources, formal leaders are threatened with loss of credibility with their departmental constituencies if they behave in a statesmanlike fashion.

At some point, however, the vice president, dean, or chair must take the strategic plan before such a group, whose members have to commit the groups that they head to support it, to agree to use it as their basis for planning, and to participate in its implementation. Governance rules may also require that the strategic plan be submitted to a faculty senate or to the faculty as a whole at some point. Such a meeting must be planned, however, so there are no surprises for either the faculty or the leader.

The executive also has an informal role in the planning process: to make sure that he or she remains the identified client in planning; to make sure that there is continuity of effort; to emphasize that objectives are implementable; to make sure that the process is credible, that it deals with problems that are real and not troublesome to the implementers; to keep people aware of interim progress; to see that one outcome is a detailed time schedule and a resource schedule (including a budget) for implementation; and to remind people that planning is an iterative process, not a linear one.[21]

A useful way to do this is to draw up a sketchy initial plan, a rough idea of where things are headed, and to present it to key people to look at, a little like the use of the "trial balloon" in politics. If no one spots a fatal flaw and people are generally positive, planning can go forward again in more depth, but not necessarily in full detail. Perhaps at the third or fourth iteration, the final details emerge, after suspicions have been dispelled in the first round or two and in enough detail to convince the doubtful that the plan is feasible and desirable.

## Linking Planning to Control and Evaluation

The planning process should take account of later needs for control and evaluation of the plan and its implementation. There is a dynamic tension in planning between too high a level of abstraction in order to maintain a coalition of interests and too detailed a level of planning to get something on paper. The risk of pious platitudes is greatest at the beginning. The process of planning and gaining consensus is painful, and it is easy to move objectives to even higher levels of abstraction, like "apple pie" and "motherhood," so that everyone can agree. For each objective it is useful to ask:

- How do we evaluate it in its present state? In a changed state?

- How do we control the situation to regulate its states?

- How do we measure the situation to identify the need for changes?

- How and when do we plan to assess success with that objective?

- What difference will it make anyway?

It is critical for those involved to know these measures, the alternative(s) generated and discarded, the key assumptions used in comparing alternatives that are considered, and the degree of certainty behind each choice. If you flipped a coin, let them know, rather than leave them puzzling over what subtleties motivated your choices.

At some point, individual objectives and their associated policies and constraints must be aggregated into an overall plan with budgets; an organization structure; manpower and training plans; equipment, materials, and space; policies on the services to be provided, including quantity, quality, and levels; and expected performance levels. Not all will be developed in detail. Some will merely be sketched out. The decisions as to the depth of detail will depend on the planning resources available, expected rates of change, degrees of consensus, and regulatory and budget process requirements.

The planner-in-chief should include planning for management and operational control in the future in the planning process. This should include how senior executives will use the plan behaviorally for reviewing presentations and proposals; the process for budget submissions and approvals; the process for manpower control, selection and rewards; and the process for replanning.

## Procedures for Setting Priorities

There are many techniques available for clarifying goals and setting priorities. In most of them, a group of knowledgeable individuals generates a list of items to which priorities are to be assigned. The list can be developed face-to-face, in a group, or separately using the Delphi or nominal group techniques to avoid dominance by a few individuals. The developed list of priorities should be disseminated widely for comment and "buy in." Often, a two-stage process is used to assign actual priorities. At the first stage, a select group reduces the list to a reasonable size. Staff or faculty then receive feedback from that process and express their preference rankings within the list.

Ruma[22] suggests a two-stage priority-setting process to determine the sequencing of change efforts. He suggests classifying organizational areas or programs in two classifications: effective/not effective (strong/weak) and amenable/not amenable to change. The bulk of the organization's effort should be focused on areas that are not effective and are amenable to change. Effective areas, especially areas that are not easily amenable to change, should be monitored to see that they remain effective. A shift there could be damaging if not prepared for.

If the organization chooses to work on the areas that are not effective and not amenable to change, the leadership should hold expectations of results to a realistically low level. Ruma further suggests that the executive then rank order the areas that are ineffective and amenable to change according to two criteria: importance and readiness for change. He suggests that management should ensure early successes by starting work with the items that are very much ready for change and, if possible, important. With a few winners under its belt, the organization will then feel confident about tackling the less tractable problems.

## Dealing with Problems with Limited Resources
In the past, academic medical centers have had relatively easy access to resources. Today that is less and less the case. Although the rewards of planning have always been high, they are now outweighed by the penalties for poor planning. Now is the time to proceed with effective planning, using a realistic set of steps, namely:

1. As a leader of an institution or a subunit, think through how planning responsibilities are to be discharged. This implies a strategy for planning and implementation based on your knowledge of the individuals involved, their roles and their relationships.

2. Be emphatic about explicitly examining and stating institutional missions and objectives and work to heighten awareness of them in everyone's minds.

3. Use analyses of the environment to guide the planning and implementation processes. Asking who is to make use of planning outputs and why and how these persons will be induced to do so are questions that will focus thinking into a strategic framework.

4. Strive for a balance between crisis management and planned change. Crisis management skills are useful in situations that must be addressed reactively. Each time the organization survives an unanticipated stress, however, a searching case review is in order to see how such crises might be avoided in the future. One might almost think in terms of an administrative clinical pathological conference.

5. Plan for critical points at which to pause and take stock. Faculty retreats need not be pleasant house parties. They can be stimuli to initiate or refocus a planning effort. Every significant leadership change creates a period of anxiety that is a fertile period for reassessing the strategy.

6. Take steps to link strategic decisions to the management control process and in some cases to operational control procedures. The strategy must be reflected and reinforced by the budget process; by performance evaluation; through hiring, promotion, tenure and pay decisions; and by grants sought.

7. As a leader, remember the aphorism attributed to Pasteur: "In fields of observation, chance favors only the mind that is prepared." Opportunity is most effectively exploited by the prepared organization, one that is alert to continually shifting interactions between institutions, technology, environment, resources, clients, and personnel.

8. Above all, the leader who undertakes to plan for an organization as diverse and diffuse as an academic medical center must have the ego strength and the tenacity to see the task through to its completion, despite many attractive intellectual distractions. This "will to manage" is a vital ingredient of successful strategic management.[5]

Consider both the benefits and risks of starting a planning process. The benefits of sound planning are great. They include more effective resource allocation and use, less crisis management, reduced interpersonal conflict because individuals understand the origins of many situational conflicts, greater support for institutional purposes, and a heightened sense that the organization and its people influence their destinies. The costs, in addition to time and energy, include conflict with those who do better in the absence of plans—the frontier cowboys, the crisis manipulators, the entrenched fiefdoms. Situational conflict will also be heightened if the organization takes off in new directions. The greatest risk, however, is in a crisis of rising expectations. People may participate in the process and expect their fantasies to be realized. Such problems will wane as people go through successive planning experiences. It is important, therefore, to remember Ruma's warning to concentrate on issues that are amenable to change and, where less tractable problems must be addressed, to communicate what little change can realistically be expected.

## Marketing

### Timing and Communications
As the planning process proceeds, the persons involved have to recognize how their methods of communicating influence the success of their work. Marketing and implementing the plan internally will be easiest if those most affected feel that they had significant input into defining objectives and that they were as informed as or more informed than those equally or less affected. This is especially true for those whom the planning process threatens with a loss of power and influence.

All individuals involved in the planning process must understand the importance of the timing of dissemination of information. This will be a delicate maneuver. Openness and candor are attributes of the trust that must be earned and maintained. Yet participation in the process clearly must be limited to those who are not gossips and who understand that information will usually be most effective if allowed to move down the chain of command. In the meantime, the rumor mills will grind away in the absence of real information. The point here is that planners must recognize that all communications, formal and informal, have the power to influence acceptance and performance.

### Strategic Marketing and Planning Activities
There is a broad array of activities that can be included under the rubric of strategic market planning. Zallocco and Joseph[25] have suggested a taxonomy that includes (1) environmental analysis, (2) business definition and mission statement,

(3) objectives and strategy development, (4) tactics, and (5) budget and control mechanisms. While they were speaking solely in terms of hospitals, these same categories also apply to the educational and research elements of the academic medical center. It is just as important to know how the funding agencies view the research image of the medical school faculty as it is to know the satisfaction of clinic patients.

### Environmental (Market) Research
The academic medical center should start its search for a strategy with analyses of its constituencies. A major tendency of academic institutions is to look inward rather than outward, to expect its "experts" to define the "needs" of the public. Drucker[24] points out that the ultimate test of any private or public organization's right to survival is its ability to meet the perceived needs of a public for service. The academic medical center will ultimately stand or fall on its ability to meet the demands presented to it. A key test of the practicality of the planning process is whether or not it gives a high priority to matching the activities planned to the potential resources available, and this includes the resources the public makes available to it.

The first step is to determine the "image" of the institution among its various publics, as well as their aspirations for it. Marketing studies show that word of mouth is the primary means people use to form opinions about professional services. Focus groups can provide an effective initial way of getting at the images and expectations that are out there. For example, the various publics include potential patients, referring physicians, faculty peers, community influentials, potential students and their parents or sponsors, alumni, staff influentials, regulators, and payers. An academic medical center is characterized by high technology, high cost, learners delivering care, and research. What are these factors doing to public perceptions and public choices? What are they doing to the resources that are available to them (students, residents, patients, grants, philanthropy, etc.)? What would it take to change that image? What types of experiences would influence it?

Usually, the academic medical center has a built-in reputation for high-technology, state-of-the-art care. This, unfortunately, is also associated at times with less of a reputation for caring and warmth, as well as perceived high cost accompanied by high value for some situations. Learners may also represent a major hazard to patient satisfaction. Few academic medical centers admit that learners are a problem, but they may be. Media exploitation of stories of unsupervised residents working long hours have sensitized the public to the possible problems.

Image is not a single blur spread over the whole academic medical center. Various service units will have distinct and not necessarily consistent images. Smith and Clark[25] suggest that these images are complex and related to physicians, technology, care, cost, and location, but even these may differ between the institution as a whole and specific service centers. Careful assessment of each segment of the organization must be made in light of the public's or clients' perception of the services being provided and of what may be desired or expected.

Another step is to gather intelligence about the competition, their image, their strengths and weaknesses, their current and probable future plans, and their relationships with patients, professionals, and payers. There are ethical and unethical ways to gain this information, but vendors, patients, the press, regulatory agencies, surveys, and others all provide timely information ethically,[26] and it should be collected assiduously.

The fact that power is diffuse in an academic medical center also means that ownership of the processes that patients and employees experience is also diffuse. Many, if not most, systems problems affecting the patient's experiences go unresolved. Ironically, while the quality of clinical practice is generally high, the quality of patient experience is low. Active quality improvement teams are a good way to look at clients' experiences and take responsibility for making them better. Advocates of an improved patient experience are needed and should be put in place.

Market research specialists should be oriented to follow these specific issues of academic medical centers—high technology, quality of care, high cost, learners, and unresolved system problems, especially communications problems. Market research is an area of marketing that is not for amateurs or generalists. It is a highly specialized area with many techniques available. The role of management is not to design, conduct, or interpret the environmental market research. It is to make sure that strategically important issues are addressed.

### Internal Marketing
One of the key markets to be researched is one's own employees. They have to buy into strategic plans and to represent the chosen image to the public. Without a special effort, those who work at an academic health center are no more likely to know about critical health care issues than is the public at large.[27] If they do take their families to a suburban hospital instead of the place where they work, the public is quick to suspect that their employer's quality of care is poor. Internal marketing "focuses on achieving effective internal exchanges between the organization and its employee groups that are a prerequisite for successful exchanges with external markets."[28] Employees are a key constituency that should not be ignored. Communicating with them on these issues is also part of their "buying into" the strategic plans.

### Competitor Analysis
The academic medical center may or may not be the only one in town. If it is, it is still in heavy competition with other health institutions for patient revenue, and these institutions may not just be community hospitals. Freestanding surgicenters can pull high-volume elective procedures such as cataracts from a hundred miles away. The academic medical center is in serious danger of being left with only the high-uncertainty, high-cost portions of patient care, with no chance of spreading the overhead costs over a wide range of procedures. The academic medical center must view its competitors broadly if it is to avoid being nibbled to death by a wide variety of providers.

### Mission Statement and Business Definition
This key area of strategy has been discussed extensively above. We have argued that it should reflect the special social purpose of the academic medical center and recognize the need to be businesslike, but still recognize that it is not a business; it is an education, research, and service endeavor forced to run a number of businesses to pay the rent.

### Objectives and Strategy Development
Again, the sections of strategic planning discussed earlier have emphasized the need for realistic objectives within a strategic framework. The important point to

remember here is that the strategies of individual organizational units are not simply linear derivatives of the strategy at the top. The overall objective might be to be a top-ten medical school, which leads the department of medicine to want to be a top-ten department of medicine and the cardiology division to want to be a top-ten cardiology division. That leads to a planning process in which cardiology deals directly with issues of competition, strengths and weakness of tenured faculty, available capital funding, research interests and funding for those, and the realities of the patients available and levels of Medicaid reimbursement in that state. It is at the level of the division that goals and objectives really become operational and measurable.[29,30] This is one reason why participation is important, because the bulk of the operational planning needed for implementation will be done at the department and divisional levels.

### Tactics
Zalloco and Joseph[23] include advertising and promotion (including public relations) and fund-raising programs in this category. This is the area that has gotten the most attention in health care marketing. As one drives around medium-sized American cities, it is not too difficult to observe that the two biggest purchasers of billboard advertising appear to be health care institutions and breweries. Yet it is, as they describe it, a matter of tactics and not strategy.

### Budget and Control Mechanisms
Zallocco and Joseph[23] lump program evaluation and review, patient satisfaction surveys, and budget allocations for planning into this last catchall category. However, Pivnicny[31] emphasizes the importance of integrating financial and strategic planning. He suggests the development of a common planning model used by the planning and the financial staffs, with common output reports going to senior management so that they can consider the impacts of proposed plans on both the programmatic and the financial strength of the institution.

The key to control is adequate feedback, and one of the most important feedbacks today is patient and other client perceptions of the service that they are receiving. Customer surveys are the usual means of gathering such data, and the health care marketing literature is full of the tactics of developing and validating survey instruments. For the manager who is not already familiar with this literature, a place to start is Reidenbach and Sadifer-Smallwood's discussion of a health care application of a model commonly used for consumer services.[32]

## Meeting the Challenge through Strategic Planning
We need to ask the question, "What is the role of academic medicine in our national life?" The 126 medical schools that characterize academic medicine form a significant segment of the health care field. They influence American medicine, and they influence the economy of every region where they are located.

We are now beginning the fifth decade since World War II. Each period has been characterized by a particular emphasis on one aspect of the mission of academic medicine. Immediately post-World War II, the era of major support for biomedical research unfolded, stimulated by the successes of the research effort during the war. The research enterprise grew remarkably and came to dominate the activities of academic medicine. In the mid-Sixties, the federal government first began to provide support for medical education and for the development of manpower.

Undifferentiated support through formula grants for medicine and the other health professions again contributed to the growth of faculty and student body. By the mid-Seventies, reimbursement for medical care through federal programs and private insurance as an employee benefit became firmly entrenched. Initially, reimbursement was focused on inpatient care, and hospitals played a prominent role in the health care scene. Advertising became acceptable, and there was emphasis on product lines, diversification, vertical integration, and across-the-board efforts to maximize income. Physicians in the private sector as well as in academic medicine became part of this picture and began to be perceived as selfish, greedy, and arrogant by association. Academic medicine became part of the competition and marketing mentality of the Eighties.

We believe that it is now time for another course correction, and, as we have pointed out, there are signs that the orientation of academic medicine is changing. It is time for a reexamination of the role of academic medicine in society. We have spoken of renewing the social contract with the community. There is much talk these days about reorienting medical education toward the training of primary care physicians. Once more, goals have been established for the recruitment of minority students and faculty. The leadership of academic medicine must reexamine its mission in the context of the needs of society, both in the immediate community and from a broader national and even international perspective.

"Research shows that successful organizations are innovative and exceedingly responsive to their changing environments. We have urged attention to strategic planning, which implies an awareness of environmental changes as a first step. But fundamental to sound strategy is a thorough understanding of where the organization is going and what it believes it is....When the environment changes rapidly, so does the excellent organization. In fact, it should be capable of anticipating environmental changes."[33]

David Dill[34] reports that, in academic institutions, management of the culture is particularly important. He suggests that the core values of the institution must be emphasized and labels this the "management of meaning." Dill believes that the techniques of managing the meaning and social integration are the keys to effective academic managements. We believe that tradition and common values are important and would argue that it is the responsibility of leadership to articulate and present a common set of values within the organization and to present this "face" to the public on behalf of the organization. This sense of purpose and a belief in the importance and value of the work of the organization is the first step in strategic management planning.[35]

## References

1.  McLaughlin, C., and others. *Strategic Planning and the Control Processes of Academic Medical Centers: A Study Guide.* Washington, D.C.: Association of American Medical Colleges, 1979.

2.  Walker, D. *The Effective Administrator: A Practical Approach to Problem Solving, Decision Making, and Campus Leadership.* San Francisco, Calif.: Jossey-Bass, 1979, p. 187.

3.  Drucker, P. *Managing the Nonprofit Organization: Principles and Practice.* New York, N.Y.: Harper Collins Publishers, 1990, pp. 45-46,99-100.

4.  Gallagher, K., and Weinberg, C. "Coping with Success: New Challenges for Nonprofit Marketing." *Sloan Management Review* 33(1):27-42, Fall 1991.

5. McLaughlin, C. *Strategic Planning: A Study Guide*. Washington, D.C.: Association of American Medical Colleges, 1979.

6. Vancil, R. "Strategic Formulation in Complex Organization." In Lorange, P., and Vancil, R. (Eds.), *Strategic Planning Systems*. Englewood Cliffs, N.J.: Prentice Hall, 1977, p. 4.

7. Anthony, R. *Planning and Control Systems: A Framework for Analysis*. Boston, Mass.: Division of Research, Graduate School of Business Administration, Harvard University, 1965.

8. Rafkind, F. "Developing Management Leaders; An Interview with Marjorie P. Wilson, M.D." Issue Paper No. 6. Philadelphia, Pa.: National Health Care Management Center, University of Pennsylvania, 1980, p. 18.

9. Mintzberg, H. "Planning on the Left Side and Managing with the Right." *Harvard Business Review* 54(4):49-58, July-Aug. 1976.

10. Stevens, R. *In Sickness and in Health: American Hospitals in the Twentieth Century*. New York, N.Y.: Basic Books, Inc., 1989, pp. 6,362.

11. Liedtka, J. "Formulating Hospital Strategy: Moving Beyond a Market Mentality." *Health Care Management Review* 17(1):21-26, Winter 1992.

12. Lewis, I., and Sheps, C. *The Sick Citadel: The American Academic Medical Center and the Public Interest*. Cambridge, Mass.: Ollgeschlager, Gunn & Hain, 1983.

13. White, K., and Connelley, J. *The Medical School's Mission and the Population's Health*. New York, N.Y.: Springer-Verlag, 1992.

14. World Health Organization. *Changing Medical Education: An Agenda for Action*. Geneva, Switzerland: World Health Organization, 1991.

15. Johnson, D. "Core Competencies Define Medical Centers of the Future." *Health Care Strategic Management* 8(7):2-3, July 1990.

16. Bower, M. *The Will to Manage: Corporate Success Through Programmed Management*. New York, N.Y.: McGraw-Hill, 1966.

17. Beckhard, R., and Harris, R. *Organizational Transitions: Managing Complex Change*. Reading, Mass.: Addison-Wesley, 1977, p. 3.

18. Delbecq, A., and Gill, S. "Justice as a Prelude to Teamwork." *Health Care Management Review* 10(1):45-51, Winter 1985.

19. Shortell, S. "Theory Z: Implications and Relevance for Health Care Management." *Health Care Management Review* 7(4):7-21, Fall 1982.

20. Cunliff, E., and Smith, P. "Total Hospital Involvement in Strategic Planning." *Health Care Strategic Management* 7(11):13-6, Nov. 1989.

21. Roberts, E. "Strategic Planning—A Framework for Managerial Decision Making: Implementing Strategic Plans." Management Advancement Program Videotape No. 5. Washington, D.C.: Association of American Medical Colleges, 1979.

22. Ruma, S. "Strategic Planning—A Framework for Managerial Decision Making: Diagnosing Organizational Problems: A Conceptual Model." Management Advancement Program Videotape No. 6. Washington, D.C.: Association of American Medical Colleges, 1979.

23. Zallocco, R., and Joseph, W. "Strategic Market Planning in Hospitals: Is It Done? Does It Work?" *Journal of Health Care Marketing* 11(1):5-11, March 1991.

24. Drucker, P. *Management: Tasks, Responsibilities, Practices*. New York, N.Y.: Harper & Row, 1974.

25. Smith, S., and Clark, M. "Hospital Image and the Positioning of Service Centers: An Application in Market Analysis and Strategy Development." *Journal of Health Care Marketing* 10(3):13-22, Sept. 1990).

26. MacStravic, R. "The Need for Competitive Intelligence." *Health Care Strategic Management* 7(1):19-22, Jan. 1989.

27. Lee, P., and others. "Effective Internal Marketing: The Challenge of the 1990s." *Journal of Health Care Marketing* 11(2):58-62, June 1991.

28. George, W. "Internal Marketing and Organizational Behavior: A Partnership in Developing Customer-Conscious Employees at Every Level." *Journal of Business Research* 20(1):63-70, Jan. 1990.

29. Vancil, R. "Strategy Formulation in Complex Organizations. *Sloan Management Review* 17(2):1-19, July 1976.

30. McLaughlin, C. *The Management of Nonprofit Organizations.* New York, N.Y.: John Wiley & Sons, 1986.

31. Pivnicny, V. "Integrating Financial and Strategic Planning." *Health Care Strategic Management* 7(9):14-6, Sept. 1989.

32. Reidenbach, R., and Sandifer-Smallwood, B. "Exploring Perceptions of Hospital Operations by a Modified SERVQUAL Approach." *Journal of Health Care Marketing* 10(4):47-55, Dec. 1990.

33. Wilson, M., and McLaughlin, C. *Leadership and Management in Academic Medicine.* San Francisco, Calif.: Jossey-Bass, 1984, p. 345.

34. Dill, D. "The Management of Academic Culture: Notes on the Management of Meaning and Social Integration." *Higher Education* 11(3):303-20, May 1982.

35. Wilson and McLaughlin, *op. cit.,* p. 349.

*Marjorie P. Wilson, MD, FACPE, is President, Educational Commission for Foreign Medical Graduates, Philadelphia, Pa. Curtis P. McLaughlin, DBA, is Professor of Business Administration and Health Policy and Administration, Kenan-Flagler School of Business, University of North Carolina, Chapel Hill.*

# Chapter 6

# The Academic Health Center as a Tertiary Referral Center and Exporter of Expertise

*by Dale D. Briggs, MD*

The academic health center (AHC) has traditionally been a product-driven organization. It has often had the luxuries of adequate or excessive patient volume and exclusivity of some services. Competition and the inevitability of universal health financing have disturbed this complacent situation. As markets expand geographically and general hospitals develop their own areas of excellence, competition for patients will increase. To be competitive, management of the AHC must change its marketing strategy. Patients, or other purchasers, will have a choice: They will choose value and service.

A patient- or consumer-driven organization is forced to respond to external pressures in a "catch-up" posture. However, to be optimally competitive, an organization should create advantages that force competitors into a reactive position. Otherwise, hospitals and ambulatory services can expect the competition to target their most successful and profitable centers of excellence. Avenues of attack will include price, quality, and market segments (niches).

Special marketing risk groups for many AHCs include the uninsured, the underinsured, and minorities, groups that often constitute a significant portion of an institution's patient base. Often taken for granted, these groups will become valuable market segments with the inevitable implementation of some form of universal health insurance coverage. The AHC should anticipate that its competitors will show immediate and intense interest in these risk groups as health care financing converts liabilities to assets. The steady flow of the underserved from an existing referral network will diminish unless the referring physicians and institutions provide high-quality service. Failure to provide convenient access and high-quality care for referral sources will result in loss of patients to more competitive and more service-oriented physicians and institutions.

This chapter will review two diverse but complementing functions of the academic health center: to serve as a tertiary referral center and to provide support for a network of health care facilities. Concurrently, it will examine management aspects of the AHC from both business and medical perspectives. The discussion will include classical models of business planning and analysis as well as models modified by the influence of the traditional missions of the AHC: research, education, and service. Projections will be based on reasonable expectations in a rapidly evolving technological and economic environment.

## The Future of the Academic Health Center

The traditional functions of the AHC are to research, to teach, and to serve. Most nonacademic businesses generally provide only two of these functions. They may develop a product (research) and sell the product or service. They usually limit teaching to the internal environment of the company or to product support. Technical information about the product is usually deemphasized or even guarded as a trade secret or competitive advantage. Conversely, the AHC is morally bound to share the results of its research and its research financing, and its charter may require that the information be made public.

Nonmedical academic institutions usually have goals and obligations similar to those of the AHC, but they traditionally do not develop the service component as extensively as health care institutions do. For example, business and engineering schools conduct research as well as teach; however, only a few faculty consultants in these schools generally provide service.

On the other hand, the AHC must maintain an active, high-quality service component for two reasons: to train students and resident health care professional trainees and to maintain a patient base for clinical and health care delivery research.

Generally, it is prudent for a business to segment its services or products, discontinuing unprofitable ones while concentrating efforts on profitable ones. However, program requirements of the AHC might not allow this pragmatic approach. Teaching and research functions might require the retention of unprofitable activities. Rather than maintain a revenue-depleting activity, the AHC might export students or patients to another facility for essential training or services, respectively. With careful planning, it should be feasible to transfer essential but revenue-depleting activities to a collaborating medical facility and still keep these functions within the health care system network.

The AHC is a complex business functioning under the influence of a complex, evolving economy. The center's success will be directly related to its ability to adapt within this economic environment. In the past, many AHCs were financed primarily with tax revenues and/or private endowment. Income from services was coincidental and often neglected. Now, as well as in the future, the ability to compete for revenue generated from services will significantly influence a center's income. Management can expect governing boards to monitor service/revenue production more carefully.

To efficiently direct the AHC, management must formulate and begin to answer many questions:

■ What is the nature of our economy?

■ What are our missions?

■ What business (or businesses) are we in?

■ What business do we want to be in?

■ What are our products?

■ How do we develop new products?

■ How do we maintain and improve quality?

■ How do we promote our products?

■ How do we distribute our products?

■ Who is our competition?

■ Should we compete or collaborate?

■ How do we continually retrain our human resources to adapt to the changing technical and economic environments?

■ What successes are possible?

■ What failures are possible?

■ What ethical constraints guide and govern us?

## The Economics of Health Care

Knowledge is the force that drives our global economy. The AHC has an opportunity to be the hub of a health care system to distribute its knowledge for the benefit of society. Health knowledge should be assimilated, created, packaged, and distributed.

The health care system cannot afford to separate its business and medical aspects. Physicians must learn to accept the vocabulary of business. For example, referring to a patient as a "customer" is not slanderous. A skilled surgical procedure that becomes a "product" benefits the patient no less.

In the United States, the value of goods produced exceeded the value of services provided prior to the Civil War. Since then, our country has been in a service-dominated economy with the ratio of services-to-goods steadily increasing. The proportion of service that can be considered transferred knowledge, in contrast to "hands-on" service, has been increasing also. This trend has been manifested in such disciplines as law, accounting, investments, computer services, communication, and even medicine. A 15 percent portion of the GNP has been projected for health care. Some analysts have viewed this as an alarming figure. However, if the automobile industry produced the same percentage of the GNP, the stockholders would be ecstatic. Likewise, the health care industry, including AHCs, should be pleased, especially if a portion is exported, thus helping the balance of trade.

To participate in an economy effectively, management of the AHC must understand the economy's characteristics. Those characteristics are largely determined by the geographic size of the market (global) in which one participates and the primary product (knowledge) of that market.

## The Global Market

Choosing the world for a marketplace is an optimistic, yet reasonable, decision. Electronic communication via wire, fiberoptics, and satellite provides virtually instantaneous contact anywhere on earth. Some forms of medical knowledge are just as valuable to someone thousands of miles away as they are to someone in the same room. The management challenge for the AHC is to make knowledge available to those who can use it, wherever they are, and to ensure reasonable compensation for financing this service.

Technology and transportability of production are the two most limiting factors in a market. In an earlier agricultural economy, the time it took to move knowledge 100 miles was measured in days. The industrial revolution lowered the time to hours. The telegraph further decreased the time to minutes, but it still imposed a capacity limit. Today digitalization and compression of electronic information results in a global distribution time that is practically instantaneous. The geographic reality of the knowledge economy is global. It is, therefore, a complex issue for management of the AHC to decide how much of this worldwide market to pursue.

Geopolitical maps show distinct boundaries. However, a map showing economic flow and information exchange would have no boundary lines between states, nations, and other political distinctions. The borders only become distinct as material goods and people are moved across them, but boundaries are not distinct as information and/or knowledge passes in electronic or written form. An opportunity for the AHC is to use this virtually unhindered access to its advantage to gain market share and to benefit its customers. Because of the universal need for its products (knowledge), the AHC may choose the size of the market in which it participates.

## Knowledge: The Primary Product of the AHC

Knowledge is often confused with information. According to Webster's dictionary information is "intelligence communicated by word or in writing; facts or data." When information, which is a collection of data, is understood and utilized by a human being, it becomes knowledge. Computers may contain enormous amounts of data and information, but they cannot use it as humans do; computers lack knowledge.

Information is only the raw material of knowledge. It exists in a variety of storage media, such as books, journals, or computer disks. Only people can utilize information; thus only human beings possess knowledge. Knowledgeable people, therefore, become human capital and should be valued as such. Investment in people is a capital investment. Efficient utilization of this human/knowledge capital is the ultimate management task of the AHC.

Knowledge, in various forms, is the ultimate product of the AHC. If capital is "any form of wealth used for the production of more wealth," knowledge is a capital asset of the organization. To develop a "product mix," to promote it, and to be competitive, management must conceptualize this asset as well as define and distribute its components. Knowledge without dissemination has no value. The AHC must inventory its knowledge/capital (product), locate and contact those that need the expertise (market), and develop ways to deliver it (distribution channels).

Ensuring compensation for the transfer of knowledge is sometimes a problem. The technology for transferring knowledge has often preceded the mechanism and/or policy for receiving compensation for it. Influencing third- and fourth-party payers to reimburse for breakthrough advancements in knowledge and innovative mechanisms for distributing both old and new knowledge is a major financial management task for the AHC. Traditional reimbursement for services has required the physical presence of the patient and the practitioner, e.g., office visit, hospital visit, consultation, or other means of contact. In the knowledge economy, the patient and the provider can often be linked electronically in a manner that is beneficial to the patient and at the same time is cost effective. Fiscal intermediaries must be educated to recognize the value of this method of health care delivery. They should not only support it but also encourage or even require it when cost effectiveness or high-quality outcome has been proven.

## Strategic Planning

The AHC is in a unique position to develop and promote tertiary care services as "centers of excellence." Members of the staff are often aware of and may be participating in the development of new technologies. Expedient conversion from a research to a concurrent service mode may be possible. Although core personnel and equipment may be available, careful market analysis must be undertaken before committing added resources to a major clinical program.

The prudent institution will define a technology development administrator to coordinate, implement, and manage these services. Acquisition of personnel, equipment, physical facilities, financing, marketing, and continuing management is essential to the success of such a program. Scientific expertise alone will succeed only with luck or until a more efficient competitor arises.

Careful coordination and cooperation between scientific and management staff are essential for success. The skills and expertise contributed by each discipline are often beyond the understanding and/or interest of the other. However, both disciplines need to work together in order to survive in tomorrow's market.

The formation of a technology research committee will provide a forum for interchange and exploration of ideas. Realities of financing, acquisition, and amortization, as well as potential marketing techniques, should be collectively considered. New technology in health care is expensive. Unlike new industrial technology, it usually does not result in decreased unit cost. Financial success, therefore, depends on utilization of the technology sufficiently to cover costs. The AHC has the potential to supplement patient care revenues with grants, donations, and government entitlements. This competitive advantage is often negated by a higher than usual uninsured or underinsured percentage of patients than its competition has.

Academic health centers have traditionally been the technical and financial resource of last resort. Often, patients have come to the AHC because of the complexity of their medical problems or the lack of financial resources to pay for their care. However, the AHC continues to train its competition. This fact, plus increasing insurance coverage and increased competition in expanding markets, makes high-quality services imperative.

Referring physicians and institutions will form new alliances with other institutions unless they and their patients are served in an exemplary manner at the AHC. An established supportive relationship with a referring physician is the best promotional mechanism. The experience of receiving expedient and high-quality services for a patient is immeasurably more effective than other techniques used, such as letters, pamphlets, or stick-on telephone numbers.

Referring physicians and institutions are also experiencing increased competition. They are sensitive about losing patients. The AHC must give careful attention to communicating with referring physicians and to returning patients to them as expediently as possible. Referring physicians will, more than ever before, want to provide as much care as possible to support their local facilities and to protect personal financial interests. Step-down care from tertiary units should be done by the referring physician/facility as it is feasible.

Promotion of the market segment for secondary and tertiary services is different from that for primary services. Patients rarely choose the source of their secondary and tertiary care. These decisions are usually made by or with the recommendation of a physician already involved in the case. Promotion of secondary and tertiary centers will be more effective if directed to physicians, institutions, and contractual payers than to the general public. However, the image of the institution will be enhanced by public awareness of tertiary centers of excellence.

## Technology Management

The AHC should be continually looking for new technology for establishing market niches. A multidisciplinary technology research committee could be an effective instrument to initiate marketing and fiscal investigation of new therapeutic modalities. Meeting regularly, the committee would begin in-depth feasibility studies by management and related clinical specialists. Expedience in the evaluation process will usually be essential. The first participant on-line with an expensive new technology may end up being the only one in the market.

High-cost technology represents unusual financial risk. The AHC should consider establishing a position of technology manager, a person to coordinate investigation, analysis, assessment of feasibility, and marketing throughout the institution's network. The technology research committee would also serve as a professional advisory and monitoring group during both analysis and implementation phases. Coile[*] compiled a list of recent and new technologies to be considered for high-technology centers of excellence. These technologies are divided into diagnostic, therapeutic, and support categories and are predicted to be commonplace in the next five years in tertiary centers and in competing facilities.

### Diagnostic Technologies

■ Computed Tomography (three-dimensional and high-speed)

■ Doppler Echocardiography (two-dimensional)

■ Low-Osmolarity Radiographic Contrast Agents

■ Magnetic Resonance Imaging

■ Low-Strength Resonance Imaging

■ Mammography

■ Outpatient Cardiac Catheterization

■ Single-Photon Emission Computed Tomography (SPECT)

■ Tumor Markers

■ Ultrasound

■ Chorionic Villus Sampling (CVS)

■ Digital Subtraction Angiography

■ High-Speed Cine-CT

### Therapeutic Technologies

■ Balloon Angioplasty

■ Continuous Arteriovenous Hemofiltration (CAVH)

■ Cochlear Implants

---

[*] Coile, R. *The New Medicine: Reshaping Medical Practice and Health Care Management.* Rockville, Md.: Aspen Publishers, Inc., 1990.

- Gallstone Pump
- Lasers
- Lithotripsy
- Streptokinase Thrombolysis versus tPA
- Extracorporeal Membrane Oxygenation (ECMO)
- Gallstone Lithotripsy
- Hyperthermia for Tumor Treatment
- Implantable Cardioverter/Defibrillator
- Percutaneous Automated Diskectomy
- Photoradiation Therapy (Photochemotherapy)

### Support Technologies

- Information Systems
- Home Care Technologies
- Personal Emergency Response Systems
- Electronic Imaging Transmission (Teleradiology)
- Digital Image Management Systems and Optical Disk Storage
- Bedside Computer Terminals

Cautious feasibility analysis of each modality will be necessary before committing to the usual high-revenue consumption of these types of projects. Pressure to implement a favored modality may be intense from interested clinical staff members. Coventuring may be an effective method to ease this pressure, to decrease financial risk to the institution, and to bring reality to the evaluation process.

## Marketing Strategies

### Collaboration
Sometimes, the formation of an alliance with a competitor is a more efficient strategy than continuing to struggle for a market share. If the market is too small to support two or more participants, each one may lose. Collaboration allows competitors to divide up failing services, allowing them to become profitable in one institution or the other. Each has then developed a strong department that should be profitable. However, careful attention must be given to the avoidance of antitrust violations in these types of arrangements.

### Networking
The AHC, because of its diverse roles and responsibilities, may not be able to divest itself of some services, even unprofitable ones. Networking with other health care facilities is a means to increase patient volume and sustain a weak service. As small and/or isolated hospitals withdraw from full service and seek market

niches, they will need referral sources for the functions they discontinue. Having an alternate source will satisfy the referring hospital's need to provide continuing care as well ensure full service for managed health care contracting. Network development can be approached from both geographic and intensity of service concepts. Ideally, both avenues should be undertaken concurrently.

### Local networks
Local networks of hospitals plus other freestanding facilities and their medical staffs are aligning to become more competitive and comprehensive in the medical marketplace. The AHC should take the initiative to form its own hub-and-spoke network. Local networks will consist of hospitals, ambulatory centers, group practices, and preferred medical specialists. Managed care contracting, access to discount purchasing, and patient referral for specialty services are common reasons for having cooperative agreements. The AHC may support the small and/or rural hospital by offering financial services, sophisticated medical information systems, marketing, and other management functions, as well as secondary and tertiary clinical support.

### Regional networks
Regional networking originated as group discount purchasing ventures. The AHC should optimally utilize this type of alliance to develop markets for its tertiary and other referral services. Regional hub-and-spoke networks are formalizing clinical relationships to ensure and direct secondary and tertiary care patients. Regionally distributed managed care plans are also evolving from these arrangements.

### National networks
National networks are developing with functions similar to those in regional networks. Purchasing clout is, of course, increased with increased group size. From a clinical standpoint, national organizations represent an excellent opportunity for the AHC to reach a broad market for its high-technology, niche services with minimal promotional expense. Prearrangement also ensures financing and increases the likelihood of stable patient census patterns.

### Global networks
Global networking is a reality in this age of instantaneous worldwide communication and jet travel. International marketing offers unique opportunities for expansion of tertiary services. These opportunities are accompanied by unique management challenges. It is relatively easy to export knowledge electronically or even to send a consultant out of the country. The importation of a patient, especially a sick one, poses greater problems. The technicalities of international travel (e.g., visa or passports) are complicated when the traveler is ill. Innovative negotiations with custom authorities, and maybe political intervention, may be necessary to expedite patient transfer across national borders. Prearranging financial details of reimbursement may prevent potentially disastrous fiscal consequences.

International marketing will, in acute cases, depend on the availability of adequate patient transport. Specialized transport services are appearing and may obviate the need for developing "in home" transport for international patients. On the other hand, it may be practical for large networks to develop transport as a viable market niche.

## Product Development

### Research as a Product

Basic science and clinical research have been the academic base of the AHC. Research attracts revenue and personnel and develops academic stature. In the new medical economic milieu, research can be expanded as a marketing and finance tool. Opportunities should be explored for private research contracting. For example, private industry and government seek expertise in exploratory ventures. Direct revenue production, as well as secondary gains in personnel, equipment, and space, may result from this type of enterprise.

The opportunity for managerial research should not be ignored. Innovative methods of health care management, financing, and delivery should be expected by-products of the AHC. Strategic use of these innovations should be valuable tools in strengthening facility network relationships.

### Management as a Product

The crisis in health care finance in this country presents many opportunities to develop management contracting as a business niche of the AHC. These are some of the factors causing financial problems in health care:

- The United States and South Africa are the only developed countries in the world without some form of universal health financing.

- Expenditures for health care approach $700 billion in this country, more than 12 percent of the GNP. Expenditures are expected to reach $2 trillion (15 percent of the GNP) by the turn of the century.

- Nearly 35 million people have no health insurance.

- Our population is aging and will require more health care.

- The cost of health care is a primary domestic concern of voters.

- The cost of health care administration as a percentage of expenditures is about double that of Canada or Japan.

- Expenditures per capita are less in many countries where citizens enjoy better health than people do in the United States.

These problems and concerns promise years of both turmoil and opportunity in the health care industry. The AHC is in a unique position to develop opportunities from this medical economic confusion.

The full-service AHC has the basic resources in personnel, facilities, and equipment to be innovative in the development of management techniques to begin solving these problems. Funds for health care delivery research may be more readily available than those for scientific research for some time. This type of research will investigate financing and reimbursement mechanisms, delivery systems, and outcomes management. Each area contains many opportunities for investigation and evaluation.

### Contracting as a Product

The delivery of health care is being changed by numerous companies providing contract management services. They are developing and selling franchise programs that license hospitals to use brand names and generic advertising. In 1988, about 2,000 facilities contracted for a variety of administrative, support, service, and clinical functions. All types of facilities contract for services, including hospitals, ambulatory centers, home care, and extended care. The contract management services for health care institutions shown in the table below have been identified.

| Growth Markets for Contract Management Services[*] | |
| --- | --- |
| **Established Contract Management Services** | **Emerging Contract Management Services** |
| Full-service management | Task-oriented management |
| Bundled management services | Unbundled management services |
| Department management | Department management |
| Housekeeping | Physical therapy |
| Food service | Gourmet food service |
| Laundry | Rehabilitation |
| Plant maintenance | Risk management |
| Biomedical engineering | Information systems |
| Pharmacy | High-tech home health |
| Emergency | Obstetrics |
| EEGs | Mobile diagnostic imagining |

[*] Coile, R. *The New Medicine: Reshaping Medical Practice and Health Care Management.* Rockville, Md.: Aspen Publishers, Inc., 1990.

The AHC should seek out and fill gaps in these services and should consider becoming competitive in established ones. Developing contractual arrangements is an excellent mechanism to solidify and expand a network of referring institutions. Successful products may be marketed and licensed to out-of-area hospitals for management fees and royalties.

Contract management of clinical services is an expanding area of opportunity for research and business development for the AHC. Approximately 20 clinical services are now available from contract firms. Among the available services are nursing, pharmacy, physical therapy, cardiopulmonary diagnostics, and intravenous nutrition. Emergency service is the most commonly contracted clinical service, with about 700 hospitals participating. Low profitability of freestanding ambulatory centers has stimulated acquisition and management contracting for these facilities. Providing these services for network hospitals could be a relationship-solidifying strategy for the AHC. Participating in ambulatory facility management becomes more of a political liability, the closer one gets to home. Care must be taken to avoid antagonizing the medical staff of the parent institution by giving the appearance of direct competition.

## Quality Improvement as a Product

The delivery of high-quality medical care has changed from an altruistic goal to a measurable management function required for accreditation by the Joint Commission on Accreditation of Healthcare Organizations (JCAHO). Implementation and documentation of interventions to improve care have become significant consumers of managerial resources. Some institutions have specialists assigned exclusively to quality improvement activities. Quality improvement standards to be required by the JCAHO in 1994 are comprehensive and may strain the capability of smaller institutions.

Outcomes management will track and intervene to improve the results of health services. Monitoring of individual practitioners, as well as of institutional departments, will be required. The managerial, clinical, and information system requirements will be significant. Quality improvement and outcomes documentation will also be necessary for effective managed health care contract negotiations.

Implementation of the principles outlined in this chapter will allow the AHC to enjoy numerous, advantageous, and profitable alliances. Win-win scenarios include the following:

- Participating in facility and professional networks on several levels to solidify patient referral patterns, thus ensuring high quality, cost containment, and mutual support of the affiliated institutions and physicians.

- Maintaining a viable primary and secondary patient base to support basic missions and to help sustain tertiary services.

- Monitoring new technology for possible implementation.

- Expanding research philosophy to include managerial and health care delivery research, quality improvement, and contract research for private business and government.

- Providing teaching functions to other institutions not only as continuing professional education but also as health management education.

- Participating in and developing managed care concepts while doing concurrent health care delivery research, including network partners when practical.

- Providing professional and managerial contracting to other facilities.

- Influencing proper reimbursement for new technologies and innovative health care delivery.

- Developing quality improvement parameters and using them to support and solidify network partners.

- Using a central information system to monitor clinical and managerial functions precisely, offering these services to network members.

- Serving as a "one-stop" market for those services needed by small and isolated facilities in order to remain viable health care units in their local communities.

As the center of a geographic health system, the academic health center has important relationships with other providers for referral purposes and with outlying communities for support services. It should not take these relationships for granted but should nurture them to protect its position in this complex, competitive environment. In addition, if the AHC plans to participate in the global market effectively, it should keep abreast of technological advances and economic changes worldwide. In order to compete nationally and even internationally, the AHC should determine which marketing strategies will accomplish its goals cost effectively and which products will offer the most opportunities for development.

## Acknowledgments

The author would like to thank Dr. Robert A. Fiser for his critical review of this paper and Marjorie McMinn for her editorial assistance.

## Bibliography

Beckham, J. "Tools for Staying Ahead in the Nineties. Part 1." *Healthcare Forum Journal* 34(3):84-90, May-June 1991.

Beckham, J. "More Tools for the Nineties. Part 2." *Healthcare Forum Journal* 34(4):63-6, July-Aug. 1991.

Cleveland, H. *The Knowledge Executive: Leadership in an Information Society.* New York, N.Y.: E. P. Dutton, 1985.

Cleverley, W. *Essentials of Health Care Finance.* 2nd Ed. Rockville, Md.: Aspen Publishers, Inc., 1986.

Crawford, R. *In the Era of Human Capital: The Emergence of Talent, Intelligence, and Knowledge as the Worldwide Economic Force and What It Means to Managers and Investors.* New York: Harper Collins, 1991.

Day, S., and others. "Pediatric Interhospital Critical Care Transport: Consensus of a National Leadership Conference." *Pediatrics* 88(4):696-704, Oct. 4, 1991.

Drucker, P. *Managing in Turbulent Times.* New York, N.Y.: Harper & Row, 1980.

Hisrich, R. *Marketing.* New York, N.Y.: Barron's Educational Series, Inc., 1990.

Hofreuter, D. (Ed.). *The Higher Ground: Biomedical Ethics & the Physician Executive.* Tampa, Fla.: American College of Physician Executives, 1991.

Kovner, A. "The Hospital-Based Rural Health Care Program: A Consortium Approach." *Hospital & Health Services Administration* 34(3):325-31, Fall 1989.

Lutz, S. "Rural Hospitals." *Modern Healthcare* 19(17):24-25,28-30,34-36, April 28, 1989.

Ohmae, K. *The Borderless World: Power and Strategy in the Interlinked Economy.* New York, N.Y.: Harper Collins, 1990.

Ohmae, K. *The Mind of the Strategist.* New York, N.Y.: Penguin Books/McGraw-Hill, 1982.

Perry, L. "Teaching Hospital Bids for Attention." *Modern Healthcare* 21(5):40, Feb. 4, 1991.

Popcorn, F. *The Popcorn Report.* New York, N.Y.: Doubleday & Co., Inc., 1991.

Schulz, R., and Johnson, A. *Management of Hospitals and Health Services: Strategic Issues and Performance.* 3rd Ed. St. Louis, Mo.: C.V. Mosby Company, 1990.

Thompson, J., and others. "One Strategy for Controlling Costs in University Teaching Hospitals." *Journal of Medical Education* 53(3):167-75, March 1978.

Vogel, L., and others. "The Referring Physician and the Teaching Center." *Mobius* 7(2):23-9, April 1987.

Whitcomb, M., and Myers, W. "Physician Manpower for Rural America: Summary of a WAMI Region Conference." *Academic Medicine* 65(12):729-32, Dec. 1990.

Zuckerman, H., and others. "The Strategies and Autonomy of University Hospitals in Competitive Environments." *Hospital and Health Services Administration* 35(1):103-20, Spring 1990.

*Dale D. Briggs, MD, is Associate Professor of Pediatrics, Section of Ambulatory Pediatrics, Department of Pediatrics, University of Arkansas for Medical Sciences, Little Rock.*

# Chapter 7

# Medical Quality Management in Academic Health Centers

*by James E. Casanova, MD*

**H**e *who ceases to try to do better ceases to do well.*—Oliver Cromwell

## History

Quality is not a new concept to the medical or academic communities. Long before the quality revolution of the last half of the 20th Century, physicians and academicians demonstrated a dedication to truth, service, and quality that often set them apart from the norms of the day. The Hippocratic oath is one testament to this dedication. The ancient rule "Primum non nocere" (First, do no harm) is another powerful, radical statement about quality, albeit much narrower than our current thinking. In fact, the satisfaction of doing one's best appears to be a drive and a need deeply rooted in many human endeavors, although not always sufficiently cultivated.

The history of the development of quality management in modern medicine has many chapters. In 1732, Dr. Francis Clifton, an English physician, wrote that "three or four persons should be employed in the hospitals to set down the cases of the patients from day to day, candidly and judiciously without any regard to private opinions and public systems, and at the years end publish these facts just as they are, leaving everyone to make the best use he could for himself....the benefit the public will receive will vastly more than balance the expense."[1] More than a century later, a nurse by the name of Florence Nightingale forcefully advocated the basic principles of quality measurement and improvement. Seasoned by her experiences in the Crimean War, she did not fit the stereotype of the self-effacing handmaiden of the day. In the early 1860s, she wrote, "A system is required in hospitals to ascertain the duration and mortality of various diseases, to enable the value of particular methods of treatment to be brought to statistical proof."[2] Almost 50 years later, in 1910, academic medicine took steps to reorganize itself according to recommendations contained in the Flexner Report, in an attempt to manage and improve the quality of medical education, which had been in disarray.

At approximately the same time as the Flexner Report, Dr. Ernest Codman advocated the establishment of an "end result system"[3] to measure the effectiveness of medical interventions. Considered eccentric at the time, his ideas nevertheless played a role in the establishment of the American College of Surgeons (ACS) in 1913 and in ACS's creation of a set of hospital standards, published in 1918. In 1919, the results of an initial survey of 692 hospitals indicated that only 89 met these minimal standards. These shocking results led not only to the burning of the "evidence" in the furnace of the Waldorf-Astoria Hotel, but, more important, to further efforts by ACS to measure the quality of hospital care. The Joint Commission on Accreditation of Hospitals (now the Joint Commission on Accreditation of Healthcare Organizations) was the direct descendent of this effort, established in 1951 by the American College of Surgeons, the American Hospital Association, the American Medical Association, and the American College of Physicians. JCAHO has remained the major force in health care quality management. Once a lone voice, it has more recently been joined by many other organizations and interested parties.

The 1960s saw the creation of the Medicare and Medicaid programs, resulting in heightened concern about the quality of care delivered in programs financed with public funds. By 1972, professional standards review organizations were created to monitor the cost and quality of these programs. Professional standards review organizations were eventually found wanting and were replaced by the present peer review organizations. Of the many functions assigned to these organizations, quality assessment has become one of the most important. Recently, the Health Care Financing Administration (HCFA) and several peer review organizations have developed a computerized database, the "Uniform Clinical Data Set,"[4] in an attempt to more efficiently monitor the quality of care in government programs. HCFA has also begun to release annual hospital mortality data, and many states have undertaken similar efforts. The Department of Veterans Affairs and the Armed Forces have also developed formal quality management programs.

The private sector has been no less interested in the quality of medical care. Managed care delivery systems have increasingly focused on quality management along with utilization review. Contracts often detail the requirements for ongoing quality management activities by provider groups. Business coalitions and consumers alike have become increasingly sophisticated about cost and quality. Data from proprietary systems, such as MedisGroups[5] and the Computerized Severity Index[5], as well as from "home-grown" systems and government databases, have been enlisted to try to analyze the value of health care purchases.

In the past 10 years, an interesting marriage has occurred between traditional medical "quality assurance" activities and the increasingly important total quality management methods being used by industry. Quality management has in fact quite recently become the accepted religion of American industry, motivated in part by the stunning success of "Kaizen" (continuous improvement theory) and related developments in Japan. This "religion" has been guided by many prophets, including Juran,[6] Peters[7] Crosby[8], and Deming,[9] to name only a few. American statistician W. Edwards Deming is credited with engineering the stunning rise in the quality of Japanese industry since World War II. In the past decade, his approach to quality has also become a blueprint for change in the United States. Deming calls for a focus on systems rather than individuals, on continuous training, data-driven decisions, a commitment to quality management by leaders of organizations and proactive continuous improvement rather than quality control by inspection after the fact. A list of Deming's now famous "14 points" is shown in the table on page 77.

Deming's ideas have been applied with little modification to the health care setting. Berwick has shown that the traditional inspection-oriented (often considered punitive) aspects of health care quality assurance can be improved by using Deming's total quality management approach,[10,11] which emphasizes improvement of systems and builds on the medical profession's long-standing commitment to the pursuit of excellence. Donabedian,[12] another pioneer in health care quality management, has authored many scholarly works that have laid the foundation for our current understanding of this subject. In the past, high-quality medical care was often delivered *in spite of* the "system," not because of it. Our success and reputation in the past have been due to the extraordinary dedication and integrity of individual practitioners. While these attributes are still very much alive in the medical community, we now need to move on to find better, more "failsafe" ways to ensure that we are consistently able to do our very best in all aspects of patient care.

---

### Deming's 14 Points[9]

1. Create constancy of purpose for improvement of product and service.

2. Adopt the new philosophy.

3. Cease dependence on inspection to achieve quality.

4. End the practice of awarding business on the basis of price tag alone. Instead, minimize total cost by working with a single supplier.

5. Improve constantly and forever every process for planning, production, and service.

6. Institute training on the job.

7. Adopt and institute leadership.

8. Drive out fear.

9. Break down barriers between staff areas.

10. Eliminate slogans, exhortations, and targets for the work force.

11. Eliminate numerical quotas for the work force and numerical goals for management.

12. Remove barriers that rob people of pride of workmanship. Eliminate the annual rating or merit system.

13. Institute a vigorous program of education and self-improvement for everyone.

14. Put everybody in the company to work to accomplish the transformation.

---

## Academic Health Centers: Is There a Difference?

At first glance, quality management in an academic health center (AHC) appears to be no different than quality management in a "community" setting. In both environments, quality has become more important for competitive, risk management, and accreditation purposes. In both settings, health care professionals strive to provide the best care possible. Medical staff and support functions are similar in both environments. Dennis O'Leary, MD, president of the Joint Commission on Accreditation of Healthcare Organizations, has stated: "We expect academic medical centers to do what we expect everyone else to do: systematically evaluate the quality of care."[13] In fact, a recent study showed no real difference in knowledge, attitudes, or quality management programs in academic hospitals versus community hospitals.[14] Despite the many parallels between these two settings, there do appear to be specific problems, specific opportunities, and specific recommendations germane to quality management programs in an academic setting.

## Academic Health Centers: The Advantages

The traditional academic "mindset" *should* be a great advantage to quality management programs if it can be harnessed for the task. In a culture that fosters questioning, innovation, and the quest for excellence, quality improvement should flourish. This culture should make it easier for individuals to dream as well as to count beans and to try out new ideas without fear of failure. In contrast, the community physician has often lacked the time and support to be truly creative. The distractions and dynamics involved in running a successful private practice can tend to choke out innovation and risk-taking, unless special effort is taken.

It may be possible to integrate traditional forms of clinical research into the quality management process. I have seen the twinkle appear in the eyes of academic physicians as they begin to consider hospital quality management programs as a source of support for personal research plans, a virtual in-house grant. While one may find a good fit between personal interests and institutional needs, often because of the scope or the timing of projects, they do not easily fit into this dual-use construct. Sanazaro,[15] as well as Jones and Strandness,[16] have addressed this issue. Their observations include: 1) clinical research alone often does not fulfill the monitoring and evaluation requirements of the institution unless a direct link can be made to the ongoing quality of care delivered by the institution; 2) the use of data from populations outside the hospital is problematic; and 3) the subject of research must be one of the important aspects of care delineated by the institution. Jones and Strandness conclude that "only certain types of medical research will be amenable to the monitoring and evaluation process—generally, research focusing on efficacy of treatments, including the results of clinical trials, comparative outcomes studies, and studies of clinical practice patterns....more applicable to monitoring and evaluation is research that studies treatments or practice patterns for which timely corrective actions and improved care can be readily documented."[16] Thus, the marriage of clinical research to quality management is viable, but, as in all marriages, one must choose one's partner with care. JCAHO would do well to further address the issue of applying longitudinal research studies to an institution's quality management efforts. Without a doubt, quality measurement and quality improvement are ongoing at academic institutions, but they may never have been labeled as such.[17]

The constant interaction of medical students, residents, fellows, and staff in clinical care is frequently cited as a source of "built-in" peer review and quality management in the academic setting. This constant questioning and review of ongoing care by many individuals may indeed contribute to quality of care, although it has been hard to quantify and document. Managing quality of care may also be facilitated at academic centers because of easy access to technology and consultants, although access to these factors certainly does not by itself guarantee quality and carries with it additional potential problems. Academic programs can also benefit from the availability of statisticians and data processing experts. In addition, a university setting offers the opportunity to interface with many other disciplines on a regular basis. This ability to "cross-pollinate" has powerful implications. Projects developed in concert by clinicians, statisticians, industrial engineers, and business school faculty may solve problems and give birth to new processes that none of these groups could attempt by themselves. This "team approach" is in fact fundamental to our most current understanding of continuous quality improvement and total quality management in health care as well as in other industries.

## Academic Health Centers: The Challenges

Despite the advantages discussed above, quality management in the academic health center often finds itself not substantially better off than in community settings. O'Leary has stated: "Academic health care centers...probably do provide high-quality care, but it is disturbing that there is little documentation to support this observation."[13] O'Leary goes on to say: "We fully acknowledge that academic health care centers carry a broad burden. Providing high-quality research, education, and patient care is a major set of responsibilities. But these related responsibilities are separable, and the fact that one meets or exceeds educational standards does not automatically assume similar performance in providing patient care....we do nobody a favor—particularly not the academic health centers—by avoiding this issue."[13]

John Colloton, director of the University of Iowa Hospitals and Clinics, has pointed out academic medicine's changing covenant with society: "In this age of data, documentation, and outcome measures, the general public and payers for medical care are no longer willing to accept bold assertions that academic health centers are the paragons of quality. Today we must prove it....toward this end, we must begin by focusing some of our most valuable resource, academic medicine's brain trust, on these important issues. To date, our investigative energy has been targeted almost entirely on biomedical research, to the virtual exclusion of comprehensive research on the medical care system as an operating entity. Even a modest redirection of a small portion of our cerebral vigor has the potential for paying enormous dividends on many fronts...."[18]

As academic health centers take up this challenge and attempt to focus more carefully on quality management, what special issues must be addressed? Perhaps academic medicine's greatest "Achilles Heel" is Deming's first point: "Create constancy of purpose." As described in Chapter 2 of this book, academic health centers have multiple and varied purposes, including education, research, and patient care. One can easily list even more. We often allude to the role model, "triple threat" professor who is accomplished in all these areas—perhaps now an endangered species. Likewise, the medical center itself is called to be a triple (at least) threat. With so many items on the agenda, it is difficult indeed to create a "constancy of purpose." In the past, patient care and institutional management activities were often overshadowed by other more "prestigious" endeavors, particularly research. This paradigm is no longer viable. Efficient management of patient care is now required for the medical center's very survival. Wards and clinics are no longer the faculty's "hobby." The need to excel at many diverse activities is a problem peculiar to academic health centers and complicates the effort to institute a quality management program.

Another potential obstacle in the pursuit of quality management is the "organizational anarchy" that often characterizes traditional academic centers. In the academic organization, "states rights" advocates have often held sway over the "federalists." Department chairs are often quite autonomous. A powerful chair may be invaluable if this individual believes strongly in quality management. On the other hand, if the chair is a "nonbeliever," or is just too distracted by other issues, quality management may remain a malnourished orphan. Lack of a tight organizational structure may also result in fragmentation and duplication of quality management activities. Complementary efforts may be under way in various parts of the realm with no awareness by the people involved. In an academic health center, Deming's ninth point, "Break down barriers between staff areas," may be much more of a challenge than in the community hospital setting. In a university environment, politics (both academic and governmental) may also contribute to confusion. Because of the many parties with an interest in the course of the academic ship, the sailing instructions may change rapidly, and tides may be unpredictable. This situation makes long-term planning a greater challenge than it would otherwise have to be.

The academic center, by virtue of its size and hallowed traditions, may also fall victim to the same disease that is endemic among other large organizations, "fossilization." James Burke, widely respected science correspondent for the British Broadcasting System, has observed that, "by definition, the hardest thing for an institution to be is flexible and ready for change....people forget that they are limited by their own gestalt, by the box they live in, no matter how clearly they believe they see the paradigm."[19] The examples of fossilization are legion: the Swiss watch industry that did not believe the quartz movement had a future; the American automobile industry that ceased to innovate and address new customer needs; the American health care industry that thought cost-based reimbursement would go on forever.

Burke's solution to this organizational disease sounds risky: "They can invest in daydream time. Let every employee get together with a computer and database—alone, in groups, networked, however—and just play. Play is an important part of creativity—wandering through the data in an associative way, seeking links that you may not have seen before. There must surely be a risk percentage of the budget that you give to people to do nothing."[19] In the old academic paradigm, this activity is called research. In the new paradigm, quality management must also be included in this type of activity.

Overconfidence is yet another obstacle that may be faced by the academic center when developing quality management programs. In an intuitive sort of way, the academic center has been considered the supreme tribunal of quality. Quality was considered the obvious product, and it was simply a matter of how to distribute it to the rest of society. Along with this view came a certain amount of disinterest in regard to suggestions from "outsiders" on how to improve—outsiders such as JCAHO, community-based medicine, or even other disciplines or other industries. Much emphasis was placed on the "interesting case" but very little on the performance of systems and processes. The spotlight has been on the spectacular breakthrough with much less interest in the Japanese concept of "Kaizen"—continuous improvement involving innumerable tiny changes for the better. It has been easier to build windows to see and analyze the world around us than to look into mirrors. As O'Leary has observed: "I believe that these institutions do a reasonably good job of reviewing specialized cases/referable cases, the unusual disease entity, through morbidity and mortality conferences, extensive consultative services, and other activities that jointly serve the patient care and educational functions. The patients generally receive appropriate attention. But academic health centers also provide a lot of bread-and-butter care for the same types of patients you find in community hospitals. And it is not too harsh, I think, to say that in many instances there is little or no formal review of these patients. Our study indicated, in fact, that physician faculty members had minimal knowledge of the monitoring and evaluation process."[13] The challenge is to attend to the ordinary, to revel in constant incremental improvement. This often requires a new way of thinking.

A significant difference between community hospitals and academic centers is the role played by residents and fellows in academic practice. House officers directly render a large proportion of the care at an academic health center. Because of this, two factors need to be addressed. First, it may be difficult to ascertain which physician is responsible for a particular patient's care. While this may appear to be a minor problem at first glance, it often becomes a challenge. Attending physicians may change. Patients may realize only that they are being managed by "a team." This potential fuzziness about responsibility can complicate the delivery of care and the assessment of quality.

Second, because it is often residents who are on the front lines of patient care, it is imperative that they be involved very directly in any quality management program. However, this is not generally the case. Quality management programs have often bypassed the resident physician. In part, this is because they have not been viewed as "real" doctors, and, in part, it has been due to disinterest on the part of the residents themselves. They have usually not been trained to value the monitoring and evaluation process and frequently have a lack of long-term commitment to the institution. In addition, there is the problem of consistent turnover, requiring constant retraining and reeducation of new groups of residents. To the extent that residents are not brought into the process however, we continue to have a huge gap in our quality management programs.

While residents often have limited knowledge and enthusiasm in regard to quality management, it is quality-of-care issues that concern them the most should they ever become patients themselves. Asked in a recent survey[20] what fears they would have should they ever become patients themselves, the three highest responses from internal medicine residents were:

- Being cared for by inexperienced housestaff.
- Errors by hospital staff.
- Loss of control.

It is apparent that quality issues are very much on their minds, even if they tend to minimize the importance of formal quality management activities. Housestaff remain a rich source of insight and ideas that has been underutilized.

Residents and medical students are also of special importance because the academic health center has an obligation to teach these future practitioners the basics of quality management theory and application. Even if they cannot all be made enthusiastic about this subject, their success in the practice of medicine in coming decades will require a basic understanding of these principles and an ability to use it to the advantage of their patients, themselves, and the institutions for which they work. Medical residents asked to identify 20 basic terms and names from the quality management literature were only able to identify a mean of 3.5

terms per resident.[20] The term most often identified was "risk management," identified by 55 percent. A sample of other terms identified included PRO (37 percent), Deming (3 percent), and pareto analysis (1 percent).

A recent survey by Ackerman and Nash[21] of 127 medical schools with 98 (77 percent) responses showed that only 27 (27 percent) offered a course or related program in quality management. Twelve of these did not offer any credit for taking such a course. Interest in this subject has been slowly building, however. A University of Tennessee survey of residents showed that "100 percent of respondents were willing to take time from the study of their clinical specialties to study practice management topics (such as quality assurance)."[22] Concerted effort is needed to find innovative ways to address quality management in the undergraduate and postgraduate curricula. Communication is needed among academic centers to share ideas and experiences, to determine what works and what doesn't. The future of quality management in medical practice may depend on how well we teach and socialize students in regard to this subject.

Access to good data has become a basic requirement for quality management in the academic setting as well as in community practice. Expertise with computerized databases and complex analyses of data may be more available in an academic setting. However, the "anarchy factor" may play an important role here also. It is not uncommon for various academic departments to go their own way when designing and purchasing computer data systems and, by default, end up with the silicone equivalent of the Tower of Babel. Data may also be under exceptionally intense scrutiny in the academic setting—even to the point of fault. The person presenting data may become a modern-day Daniel walking into a lions' den of hungry hairsplitters. In this scenario, while good data are everyone's goal, the demand for perfect data may become an obstacle in the path of even minor accomplishments.

Academic health centers have helped to pioneer several of the severity-of-illness data systems now in use, such as MedisGroups and the Computerized Severity Index. Geehr has written a concise critique and comparison of these systems.[5] Some institutions have developed their own systems. The Medical College of Wisconsin has worked with HCFA in the development of the "uniform clinical data set" now being tested by peer review organizations as well as by one of the college's major teaching hospitals. The current focus of much quality management activity is the measurement and comparison of outcomes. Instruments to quantify quality of life and functional ability have been developed, such as OT FACT[23] and the functional screening test for the elderly proposed by Lachs et al.[24] The further development and application of user-friendly clinical databases and outcomes instruments is an important area where academic-based health services research can make a huge contribution to the field of quality management.[25] The development of practice parameters and guidelines is another fertile area, as is the development of good clinical "indicators." For example, the University Hospital Consortium has recently published a volume on clinical indicators that the group developed and tested.[26]

Several other aspects of quality management at academic health centers should be addressed. Deming's Point 7 is "Adopt and institute leadership." Because of the many claims on the time and energy of academic leaders, quality management activities run the risk of becoming a form of "scutwork" that is delegated to the most junior faculty members. However, as in nonmedical settings, such an approach invariably leads to failure. All the high priests of the quality management movement, without exception, agree: If the members of the organization do not perceive quality management as a personal and compelling interest of the organization's leaders, it is dead in the water.

Deming's thirteenth point is "Encourage education and self-improvement for everyone." Quality management cannot be done as someone's "hobby." Appropriate education is necessary. Academic health centers have traditionally taken great researchers and publishers and promoted them to management positions, often without providing the specialized training necessary for success in the new endeavor. In regard to quality management, this approach is no less short-sighted. The organization needs to identify individuals with interest and talent in quality management and have them pursue career tracks that train them and allow them to excel in this area of endeavor.

Finally, the role of the hospitals, in many instances, has been overshadowed by the role of faculties and medical schools. Hospital administration and medical staff activities may then become emasculated, even though the hospital and its governing body are responsible for the activities taking place within its walls. This situation produces a "phantom" hospital medical staff, with decreased loyalty and dedication to the hospital and its particular quality management programs. Community hospitals are blessed with not having to deal with this situation.

## Summary

Very little has been published in the literature that specifically addresses quality management at academic health centers. While quality management activities at academic health centers share much in common with such activities elsewhere, there are situations peculiar to the academic setting.

Physicians as a group have shown some reluctance to learn about and support quality management activities.[10,14] Perhaps this has been with good reason--it has often been difficult for physicians to point to concrete accomplishments or personal utility accrued from this process. In many ways, quality management has yet to prove itself useful, but in many ways it has also yet to be tried.

In summary, an action plan for implementing quality management at an academic health center should include at least the following basic principles:

■ Strive to create constancy of purpose.

■ Establish genuine support for the process at the highest levels of the organization.

■ Train appropriate individuals thoroughly; then give them time to both work and dream.

■ Use an interdisciplinary approach.

■ Marry the quality management process to health services or clinical research when appropriate.

■ Develop an appreciation for "kaizen"—slow continuous improvement vs. spectacular leaps forward.

■ Stress systems improvement over policing of individuals.

■ Develop good, user-friendly, networkable data systems.

- Avoid traditional academic organizational anarchy. Build bridges. Build consensus.
- Involve housestaff in the quality management process.
- Develop curricula in quality management at both undergraduate and graduate levels.
- Be patient. Expect delayed gratification. Appreciate small gains.

Perhaps the most significant development in quality management at this time is the emergence of "continuous quality improvement" and "total quality management" techniques (built on the Deming approach) alongside traditional "quality assurance" activities.[27,28,29,30] Quality assurance has often been viewed as bureaucratic, punitive, intrusive—even caustic. These newer approaches encourage a philosophy of improvement rather than a policing function. This is in agreement with Deming's third point: "Cease dependence on mass inspection." Quality assurance "bean counters," the data-gathering arm of quality management, are still needed, but academic physicians are much more likely to support a process that helps them dream and innovate; that helps turn good science into good service.

## References

1. Heasman, M. *SCRIPS Success or Failure in a Question of Quality?* McLachlan, G. Ed. London: Oxford University Press, 1976, p. 173.

2. Cook, S. *The Life of Florence Nightingale.* Vol. 1. New York, N.Y.: MacMillan, 1942, p. 430.

3. Roberts, J., and others. "A History of the Joint Commission on Accreditation of Hospitals." *JAMA* 258(7):936-40, Aug. 21, 1987.

4. Hutton, R., and others. *The Uniform Clinical Data Set Project.* Madison, Wis.: Wisconsin Peer Review Organization, 1990.

5. Geehr, E. *Selecting a Proprietary Severity-of-Illness System.* Tampa, Fla.: American College of Physician Executives, 1989.

6. Juran, J. *Managerial Breakthrough.* New York, N.Y.: McGraw-Hill, 1964.

7. Peters, T., and Waterman, R. *In Search of Excellence.* New York, N.Y.: Warner Books, 1982.

8. Crosby, P. *Quality Is Free.* New York, N.Y.: New American Library, 1980.

9. Deming, W. *Out of Crisis.* Cambridge, Mass.: Massachusetts Institute of Technology, 1986.

10. Berwick, D., and others. *Curing Health Care.* San Francisco, Calif.: Jossey-Bass, 1990.

11. Berwick, D. "Continuous Improvement as an Ideal in Health Care." *New England Journal of Medicine.* 320(1):53-6, Jan. 5, 1989.

12. Donabedian, A. *Explorations in Quality Assessment and Monitoring: The Definition of Quality and Approaches to Its Assessment.* Ann Arbor, Mich.: Health Administration Press, 1980.

13. Friedman, E. "The JCAH Quality Initiative: What Can Hospitals and Physicians Expect?" *Physician Executive.* 13(4):2-6, July-Aug 1987.

14. Casanova, J. "Status of Quality Assurance Programs in American Hospitals." *Medical Care.* 28(11):1104-9, Nov. 1990.

15. Sanazaro, P., and others. "Assessment of Teaching and Research as Systematic Quality Assurance." Unpublished report for the Joint Commission on Accreditation of Hospitals. Chicago, Ill., 1986.

16. Jones, L., and Strandness, D. "Integrating Research Activities, Practice Changes, and Monitoring and Evaluation: A Model for Academic Health Centers. *Quality Review Bulletin.* 17(7):229-35, July 1991.

17. Hopkins, E. "The Mortality and Morbidity Conference as a Quality Assurance Mechanism: Can M + M = M + E?" *Journal of Quality Assurance.* 11(2):10-11,36, April-May 1989.

18. Colloton, J. "Academic Medicine's Changing Covenant with Society." *Academic Medicine.* 64(2):55-60, Feb. 1989.

19. Flower, J. "Where Elephants Go to Die: A Conversation with James Burke." *Healthcare Forum Journal.* 31(2):40-5, March-April 1988.

20. Casanova, J., and Barnas, G. "Medical Residents Knowledge and Attitudes Concerning Quality Assurance." *Academic Medicine* 67(4):285, April 1992.

21. Ackerman, F., and Nash, D. "Teaching the Tenets of Quality: A Survey of Medical Schools and Programs in Health Administration." *Quality Review Bulletin.* 17(6):200-3, June 1991.

22. King, B., and others. "Internal Medicine Chief Residents Suggest Need to Improve Health Care Delivery and Public Policy Education." *IMCARE Brief.* July 1990, pp. 3-15.

23. Smith, R. *OT FACT. Software and Operating Manual.* Rockville, Md.: American Occupational Therapy Association, 1990.

24. Lachs, M., and others. "A Simple Procedure for General Screening for Functional Disability in Elderly Patients." *Annals of Internal Medicine.* 112(9):699-706, May 1, 1990.

25. Ellwood, P., and others. "The Future: Clinical Outcomes Management." In *Health Care Quality Management for the 21st Century.* Couch, J., Ed. Tampa, Fla.: American College of Physician Executives, 1991.

26. *Compendium of Clinical Indicators.* Oakbrook Terrace, Ill.: University Hospital Consortium, 1991.

27. Laffel, G., and Blumenthal, D. "The Case for Using Industrial Quality Management Science in Health Care Organizations." *JAMA* 262(20):2869-73, Nov. 24, 1989.

28. Jennison, K. "Total Quality Management—Fad or Paradigmatic Shift?" In *Health Care Quality Management for the 21st Century.* Couch, J., Ed. Tampa, Fla.: American College of Physician Executives, 1991, p. 444-64.

29. Kritchevsky, S., and Simmons, B. "Continuous Quality Improvement: Concepts and Applications for Physician Care." *JAMA* 266(13):1817-23, Oct. 2, 1991.

30. Berwick, D. "Controlling Variation in Health Care: A Consultation from Walter Shewhart." *Medical Care.* 29(2):1212-25, Dec. 1991.

*James E. Casanova, MD, is Director of Quality Assurance, Milwaukee County Medical Complex, Medical College of Wisconsin, Milwaukee.*

# Chapter 8

# Clinical Quality, Risk-Adjustment, and Outcome Measures in Academic Health Centers

*by Susan I. DesHarnais, PhD, and Curtis P. McLaughlin, DBA*

## Introduction: History, Current Interest

One issue likely to polarize the staff of an academic health center (AHC) in today's turbulent times is who should evaluate clinical performance and how. Friction arises over issues of both quantity of work performed and its quality. The issue of quantity, however, is relatively easy to address objectively. Issues of quality are much more difficult, both politically and in terms of measurement. If an academic health center is to deal with the myriad quality issues and pressures that it faces, we believe that its leaders need a number of sets of knowledge on:

■ The historical development of quality measurement in health care.

■ A conceptual framework for analysis in quality management.

■ Procedures for monitoring health outcomes.

■ An understanding of the institutional responses available for addressing quality issues in the AHC context in all legs of the "three-legged stool."

While there is much current interest in using measures of patient outcomes to evaluate the quality of clinical care, this focus is not new. In the 1860s, Florence Nightingale developed and used a systematic approach to collecting and analyzing information on differences in mortality rates across hospitals. She evaluated the effects of introducing improvements in cleanliness and nutrition on the death rates of the sick and wounded soldiers treated during the Crimean War. Fifty years later, Dr. E.A. Codman reported on his study of the end results of care in the United States. "This famous study emphasized the same issues that are being discussed today when examining the quality of care, including...the necessity of taking into consideration the severity or stage of the disease; the issue of comorbidity (two or more illnesses present at one time); the health and illness behavior of the patient, and economic barriers to receiving care."[1]

We did not, however, move in a straight path toward using outcome measures to evaluate the quality of care. Outcome measures were not used more, because there were both technical and historical/political problems. The technical problems related to data availability and data processing. In the second half of this century, it became easier to monitor the outcomes of hospital care using computers and large databases and to develop more sophisticated techniques for modeling risk factors affecting the outcomes of care. Improved access to data will be discussed shortly; however, a more basic issue will be discussed first: the politics and history of quality assessment in the United States.

### Politics of Quality Assessment

In 1913, the American College of Surgeons (ACS) was formed to develop "minimal essential standards of care for hospitals as a first step toward the provision of quality care in American hospitals."[2] The work of this group led in 1918 to the Hospital Standardization Program, which developed into an accreditation process that set minimum standards for medical staff credentialing, privileging, and monitoring functions and for adequate medical records and equipment. At that time, virtually no hospital could meet even those minimal standards, although by 1951 some 3,000 hospitals were accredited by the Hospital Standardization Program.[2]

In 1951, the Hospital Standardization Program became the Joint Commission on Accreditation of Hospitals (JCAH). JCAH, created as a private, not-for-profit, voluntary agency, assumed responsibility for the accreditation program, initially using the ACS standards. The JCAH standards were later expanded to cover administrative issues. The JCAH program gained political acceptance. Accreditation was required for licensure and Blue Cross participation in many states and eventually for participation in federal programs.

JCAH emphasized establishing a proper environment for providing high-quality care, rather than determining whether high-quality care was actually being provided. Over many years, the focus shifted from structure to process. By the 1980s, hospital quality assurance personnel were asked to identify problems, set goals, focus on errors in the process of care, and demonstrate that they had met their own goals. The standards did not, however, indicate how potential problems were to be identified or addressed. "JCAH survey results indicated that many hospitals and other facilities were focusing on issues that could be readily resolved, or that the problems did not reflect the major clinical activities of the department or service, in terms of either volume or high-risk potential. What appeared to be missing was a rational approach to identifying potential issues that would impact on patient care."[2]

Because JCAH assumed a central role in the accreditation of hospitals, many hospitals structured and focused their quality assurance activities primarily to be in compliance with the JCAH quality assurance survey/guidelines. Quality assurance was defined as a function carried out by clinicians within the hospital. The JCAH approach to quality assurance largely reflected the values of society. Since the beginning of this century in the United States, society has delegated the establishment of quality standards to the medical profession. As Starr points out, "Doctors and other professionals have a distinctive basis of legitimacy that lends strength to their authority. They claim authority, not as individuals, but as members of a community that has objectively validated their competence. The professional offers judgments and advice, not as a personal act based on privately revealed or idiosyncratic criteria, but as a representative of a community of shared standards. The basis of those standards in the modern professions is presumed to be rational inquiry and empirical evidence."[3]

Caper has summarized the effects on the medical profession of this delegation of authority: "Being the perceived custodian of its own standards has distinct advantages for professions such as medicine. First, it has permitted medical professionals to attain, and retain, a very high level of autonomy, both for themselves as a group and for their individual members. Second, it has allowed them largely to determine working conditions and terms of payment. Third, it has helped turn medical decision making into a 'black box,' relatively immune to outside examination."[4]

Much work took place in the mid-1900s in studying quality and in developing criteria, standards, and protocols, as chronicled by Donabedian.[5] In addition, a substantial amount of research occurred documenting variations in medical care practice[6,7]; unnecessary surgery[8]; and preventable complications.[9-11] These studies, along with others, demonstrated a need to monitor and improve medical care practice. There has, however, been a strong resistance by many members of the profession when it comes to measuring quality, particularly if the evaluations are performed by nonphysicians, even if the evaluators are using explicit protocols that were developed by physicians. In a recent editorial, Chassin pointed out that, "Many physicians think about quality of care the way Justice Stewart characterized his ability to recognize pornography: 'I shall not today define the kinds of material I understand to be embraced within that shorthand description [hard-core pornography]; and perhaps I could never succeed in intelligibly doing so. But I know it when I see it.'"[12] Chassin goes on to note that, "A growing armamentarium of new quality assessment tools renders this proposition dangerously obsolete."

By the 1970s and 1980s, conditions had changed. As rapid advances took place in medical technology, as the cost of medical care rose in an unprecedented manner, and as evidence began to accumulate about severe quality problems, the government and the public took a growing interest in measuring the quality of care.

During this same period, data on health care use and costs became increasingly available to consumers and regulators, as well as to physicians and hospitals. This change in data availability was significant, making it possible for both professionals and others to compare the performance of various providers.

There were a variety of factors creating a demand for and availability of data on quality, outcomes, and costs of care from hospitals and professionals:

■ A legal case (*Darling v. Charleston Community Memorial Hospital*, 1963) established that a hospital governing body is responsible for knowing about problems in patient care and the actions staff has taken to resolve problems. This case established the concept of "corporate liability, meaning that the hospital can be held independently liable for its negligence in failing to establish a system of safe practices, as defined by the industry." *Darling* generated demands for information on the part of hospital administrators and board members.

■ Corporatization of medicine: HMOs, PPOs, and franchises became much more prevalent in the 1970s and 1980s. These types of organizations demanded data on costs, use patterns, and practice patterns, because such information was crucial in managing these types of plans. It was essential to evaluate the costs and quality of care given by the providers with whom these organizations contracted.

■ Broader concern with quality in industry: Many industries in the United States became concerned with methods of measuring and controlling the quality of the products and services they produced. There was a growing focus on using scientific methods, harnessing the energy and creativity of all levels of personnel in an organization. Total quality management (TQM) principles were adopted by many U.S. industries. In many communities, industries using TQM were represented on hospital boards as well. The concepts were introduced into hospital management and eventually began to change the way certain hospitals approached quality problems.

■ Hospitals wanted quality information on physician performance for appointment and reappointment decisions. Hospitals often lacked the ability to compare physician performance in terms of outcomes produced or resources utilized. As cost containment pressures increased along with concern for quality, many hospitals wanted objective information on physician performance as part of decision-making on privileges.

■ In the more competitive climate, hospitals want information on quality and costs for planning and marketing. If a hospital knows that it is either effective or ineffective in producing certain kinds of services, it can make planning and marketing decisions accordingly.

■ Hospitals are developing information systems that integrate medical records, risk management, quality management, and financial management systems as part of a new competitive climate under the Medicare Prospective Payment System. Many hospitals are developing integrated management information systems that provide data on both inputs and outcomes for various types of patients.

■ Hospitals have become interested in measuring patient outcomes as a defense against mortality data released by the Health Care Financing Administration (HCFA). In some communities, hospitals have received publicity as having high mortality rates since HCFA began releasing such information to the public in the mid-1980s. Because the methods used to derive these rates have had flaws, in many cases the negative findings could be depicted as invalid.

■ Specialty societies wanted to set standards for certain procedures and conditions in order to ensure that good care was provided. They wanted information on variations in practice in order to identify areas where there were problems or uncertainty. Such information could then be analyzed in order to promulgate standards for better practice of medicine within the specialty. In addition, some professional societies wanted information on practice patterns for setting standards for board certification.

The increased availability of data on the use, cost, and outcomes of medical services also enabled consumers, insurance companies, and regulatory agencies to analyze trends in the use and costs of health care services independently and to draw their own conclusions.

Employers, unions, consumers, and insurance companies began to demand access to such data for several reasons:

■ Unions and industry demanded such information as they negotiated contracts. As new benefits were added, it was necessary to analyze whether they were worth what they cost. In some cases, it was necessary to evaluate the performance of providers such as HMOs in order to decide whether to offer certain plans as options to workers.

■ Companies that self-insured needed to develop information on use, costs, and outcomes in order to better manage their insurance plans. Local providers that used excessive resources or had consistently poor outcomes could pose a real problem for such plans.

■ PPO contracts also required that the contracting agency exercise care when designating preferred providers. If these providers were producing poor outcomes, marketing of the plan would be impossible, and the PPO could face legal problems.

■ Consulting firms that advised insurance companies, labor, industry, or hospitals desired good data on costs and outcomes so that they could analyze choices and provide useful information to their clients.

■ Insurance companies needed such information in order to market their products successfully in a more competitive environment.

In order to provide standardized data sets on costs and outcomes, insurance commissioners and state legislators in many parts of the country (California, Iowa, Maine, Massachusetts, New Hampshire, New York, Vermont, Washington, West Virginia, and others) mandated that hospitals report these data. Several states have prescribed the specific data elements that are required. In many cases, new data elements were mandated beyond the common data set used for billing purposes, at considerable cost to hospitals.

Federal regulators (PROs/HCFA) began to find new uses for data on cost and outcomes of medical care. The federal government used the information for developing changes in payment systems, both for hospitals (DRGs) and for professionals (relative value scales). It became clear that the federal and the state programs were paying large amounts of money for treatments and/or procedures that may not be the most effective way of caring for patients. By the 1980s, the federal government allocated research dollars for "effectiveness research" to learn more about the most effective treatments in areas where great variations in medical practice were discovered.

Also, consumers began to take a much more active role in their own health care. The "women's movement" in the 1960s and 1970s emerged as a force that was critical of many medical practices. Other consumer interest groups also came forth to question the effectiveness of various practices. Individual consumers, as they had to share costs, get second opinions, select providers from panels in HMOs, and make decisions concerning treatment options, became interested in obtaining accurate and useful data on costs in relationship to the outcomes of care.

Interest in evaluating the quality of care thus moved from the professional domain to the public domain. The medical profession was under attack from the outside, as government and consumers sought to measure and evaluate quality. In particular, these groups sought to measure the value received for their money, to evaluate the relative effectiveness of various treatments, and to compare the quality of care provided by different hospitals.

This interest led to or paralleled the development of more sophisticated, complex, and useful models of medical decision-making, including computerized decision-making systems, complex treatment protocols for various diseases, and risk-adjusted measures of hospital performance.

## Framework for Quality Management

### Definition of Quality

Quality may be defined in many ways and from many perspectives. The Office of Technology Assessment defined quality of care as "the degree to which the process of care increases the probability of outcomes desired by patients, and reduces the probability of undesired outcomes, given the state of medical knowledge."[13]

Donabedian has observed that definitions of quality ordinarily reflect the values and goals of the current medical care system and of the larger society of which it is part.[14] He distinguished several aspects of care that one might choose to measure[15]:

■ **Structure**, the resources available to provide health care.

■ **Process**, the extent to which professionals perform according to accepted standards.

■ **Outcome**, the change in the patient's condition following treatment.

In addition, he defined quality broadly, to include not just technical management, but also management of interpersonal relationships, access, and continuity of care.

One can assess and measure quality using Donabedian's concepts and models, as presented in the matrix in figure 1, below, as a framework. Within each square of the matrix, one can define aspects of quality for which criteria and standards can be developed. For example, under "structure/accessibility," one might measure the scope and nature of services provided, provisions for emergency care, or geographic factors, such as distance. Within "technical management/process," one might measure the adequacy of diagnostic work-up and treatment for a particular condition.[15] The value of this matrix is that it helps us to define quality broadly and to identify the components that we might wish to measure throughout the academic health center.

| Figure 1. Matrix for the Measurement of Quality[15] | | | |
|---|---|---|---|
|  | Structure | Process | Outcome |
| Accessibility |  |  |  |
| Technical Management |  |  |  |
| Management of Interpersonal Relationships |  |  |  |
| Continuity |  |  |  |

Why might one choose to monitor structure, process, *and* outcomes? There are advantages and disadvantages to using each of these approaches. It is relatively simple to monitor structure. In many cases, one can simply do an "inventory" using a checklist. JCAH took this approach in its early days, because there was some agreement that certain structural elements were needed as minimal standards to ensure an environment in which good care was possible. It is obvious, however, that adequate structure does *not* ensure good outcomes.

Process measures take into account professional performance and would seem to be more closely correlated with better outcomes. It should be obvious, however, that outcomes are not determined solely by professional performance. Other factors, such as the patient's condition at the time of treatment, patient compliance, patient age, and chance also enter into the equation. Nevertheless, it is often easier to measure provider performance than it is to measure patient outcomes for many diseases. One can use process measures to determine whether the professional has performed adequately *for those conditions where there is substantial agreement* on what constitutes "acceptable" care and where the technology is reasonably effective.

Health care leaders would also like to monitor the outcomes of care, to measure the effect the treatment has had on the patient's condition. It should be noted, however, that it is much more difficult to measure outcomes than it is to measure structure or process. Ideally, one would like to obtain data on patient health status before and after treatment for a large national sample of hospitals. Instead, we usually end up measuring variations in rates of adverse consequences of treatment across hospitals, under the questionable assumption that hospitals with the lowest rates of adverse events are producing better patient outcomes.

To construct measures of hospital outcomes, two separate but related problems must be solved: how to take into account differences across hospitals in the types of patients treated, and how to take into account differences in the severity of illness in the patients treated across hospitals. These issues will be discussed in more detail below.

## Procedures for Monitoring Outcomes

Criteria and standards must be developed in order to monitor outcomes. Such standards may be developed in three different ways:

■ **"Absolute" (Normative): Efficacy as determined by clinical trials and/or consensus conferences.** Standards developed in this manner by academic health centers reflect the ideal practice of medicine, or the best possible outcomes that can be achieved under optimal circumstances, i.e., the most skilled surgeon, the best possible equipment, and the best trained team assisting. While it is useful to know the theoretical "efficacy" of a treatment, or the best possible results one could achieve, such standards may not be realistic under ordinary circumstances of practice.

■ **Empirical: Relative to other institutions treating similar patients.** Standards developed by comparing oneself to other institutions treating similar patients may be useful to help identify problem areas. If, for example, a hospital is experiencing 20 percent more unanticipated readmissions than other hospitals when treating a specific type of patient, that could be a signal that some correction is needed. On the other hand, it is possible that the "average" care in the community is poor. Such comparisons are only relative to the level of quality in the institutions used for comparisons.

■ **Institutional approaches, based on self-comparisons over time.** Such standards are often used in conjunction with total quality management/continuous quality improvement. One collects observations of the same phenomenon over time, to determine if a process is in control (small random variations) or out of control (major fluctuations). This information uses the institution as its own "control," with the goal of continuously raising standards in the institution. While this approach is useful, some external comparisons are required to understand how to prioritize problems. One needs such external comparisons (benchmarks) to decide which processes to address first.

### The Need for Risk Adjustment

Although mortality rates and measures of adverse events are potentially useful to providers and possibly to patients as one way to measure quality of care, such information can be misleading and potentially damaging if misused. This is particularly important when considering how such "report cards" might be used by the government or the public. Such information must be compiled and interpreted correctly. It has been demonstrated in several studies that raw death rates, without adjustment for differences in case mix and case complexity, lead to misleading comparisons among hospitals, with those hospitals that treat "riskier" patients appearing to provide poorer care.[16-19] These findings demonstrate clearly that death rates must be risk-adjusted and interpreted carefully along with other indicators of quality. This is especially important to academic health centers, with their tendency to receive the cases with the highest risk and complexity, either through referral networks or through dumping.

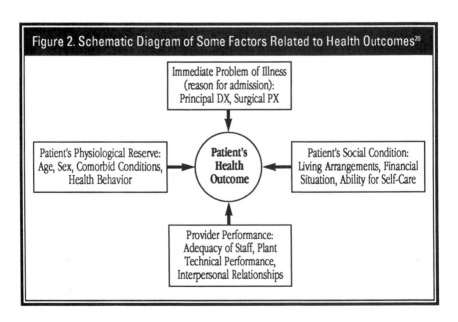

Figure 2. Schematic Diagram of Some Factors Related to Health Outcomes[20]

Immediate Problem of Illness (reason for admission): Principal DX, Surgical PX

Patient's Physiological Reserve: Age, Sex, Comorbid Conditions, Health Behavior

Patient's Health Outcome

Patient's Social Condition: Living Arrangements, Financial Situation, Ability for Self-Care

Provider Performance: Adequacy of Staff, Plant Technical Performance, Interpersonal Relationships

In a general sense, differences in outcomes across hospitals (patients' responses to treatment) can be viewed as a result of several different factors that may influence health outcomes. Figure 2, page 94, illustrates that this is a complex situation. To measure the effect of provider performance on outcomes with accuracy, it is necessary to control for all the other factors. This is clearly not possible, given the existing data sets and measurement tools. However, because "report cards" on providers are going to be produced, it is essential to try to develop as valid an approach as possible for risk adjustment.

Historically, two different approaches have been used to perform risk adjustment of hospital mortality data: hospital-level variables to adjust crude death rates and indirect standardization of patient-level data. Hospital-level data were used in several early studies. In the study by Roemer et al.,[21] hospital-level aggregate measures of patient characteristics (e.g., average age, percentage nonwhite, and percentage of cancer deaths), along with hospital characteristics (e.g., control, occupancy rate, and technology level), were modeled in an attempt to understand whether these proxies for case mix and case complexity were related to the observed differences in crude death rates among hospitals. They reasoned that if these hospital-level proxy measures were related to the crude death rates, they could be used to adjust the rates more accurately to represent each hospital's performance.

This early risk adjustment, as the authors acknowledged, was rather crude. They justified the approach by pointing out that detailed patient-level data on diagnosis and severity of illness were then not available. Therefore, they used hospital-level proxy measures as an indirect approach to estimating case mix and case complexity. The authors stated: "Ideally, one would like to examine the exact diagnosis of each patient admitted and classify it according to a scale of gravity, which might be based on case fatality rates derived from a general literature of clinical investigation....But it is obvious that such a task of calculating average case severity by such an analytic process could present formidable problem of data collection."[21] It certainly would have been difficult in the 1960s, given the limited availability of computers, to model the risks of death for all types of hospital patients using large data sets, even if such information had been available.

Because hospital-level data are of limited use as proxy measures to account for differences in case mix and case complexity across hospitals, there is no apparent reason to use hospital-level data today. Discharge-level data are now available and are much more sensitive for measuring differences in case mix and case complexity across hospitals. The techniques of using adjusted discharge-level outcome data are documented in early studies, such as the National Halothane Study in the 1960s,[16] the Stanford Institutional Differences Study in the 1970s,[22] and work by Luft on the relationship of surgical volume to mortality.[23] In an article summarizing many of the methodologic issues in the risk adjustment of outcome data, Blumberg described indirect standardization, the principle technique used for risk adjustment of discharge-level data: "Indirect standardization is the method most widely used for risk-adjusted outcome studies. It requires estimates of the expected outcome in a study population, based on the outcome experience of a standard population. To estimate expected outcome, the numbers of cases in the study population with risk-related attributes are multiplied by the probability of the outcome in a standard population with matching attributes. These expected outcomes in the study population are then compared with the observed number having that outcome in the same study population....The first step involves the development and testing of a risk-prediction model, while the second step is a study of the residuals of the observed less the expected outcomes in the study population."[24]

Eight recent risk-adjusted outcome studies are summarized in table 1, below. The scope of these studies was limited to very specific types of cases, except for the study by Hebel et al.,[25] which was comprehensive, insofar as it included all types of hospitalized patients. However, the database used by Hebel et al. for indirect standardization was limited to four hospitals in one community. Large and representative data sources are essential if indirect standardization is to be valid. Each study in table 1 used a different set of variables for risk adjustment. Age was measured in various ways and was found to be significant in predicting risk of death in all the studies. Other factors, such as emergency status of the patient when admitted, race, sex, and Medicaid (as a proxy for poverty), were used in some of the studies to predict risk of death.

| Reference Number | Data Source | Scope | Adjustment Variables | Iatrogenic Disease |
|---|---|---|---|---|
| 7 | Prospectively collected from 9 pediatric ICUs in teaching hospitals | Pediatric ICU patients | Age, clinical service, emergencyor scheduled, Physiologic Stability Index Score | Excluded |
| 19 | Prospectively collected from 13 tertiary ICUs | ICU patients | APACHE II scores | Excluded |
| 26 | CPHA | Seven surgical procedures | Age, sex, LOS, procedure-specific indices of severity, multiple vs. single dx, operation within 6 hours, payer | Included in multiple dxs |
| 23 | CPHA | Cardiac catheterization | Age (3 groups), dysrhythmia (Y,N), heart failure (Y,N), other single secondary dx, multiple secondary dx (Y,N) | Included as any other secondary dxs |
| 22 | CPHA and chart reviews and patient and provider interviews from 17 hospitals | 15 surgical categories | Physical status apart from principal disease, stage, age, sex, emergency status, cardiovascular status, interaction terms | Excluded |
| 27 | Medicare claims (Maine) and provincial claims (Manitoba) | Prostatectomy (population approach) | Previous history of hospital/ SNF treatment, age, type of operation, secondary cancer, secondary cardiovascular, secondary other | Included as secondary dx |
| 28 | NCHSR (HCUP) | Four surgical groups | Age (five groups), sex, stage, number of dxs, Medicaid or no insurance (Y,N) | Included as number of dxs |
| 25 | 100 percent of hospital records from four hospitals (all in one city) | All cases in four hospitals | Age, race, sex, payer, 83 MDCs, any secondary diagnoses (Y,N), any surgery(Y,N) | Included in secondary dxs |

Table 1. Examples of Recent Outcome Studies Based on Patient-Level Data

One of the more difficult problems each of these researchers faced was how to define operationally the severity and the complexity of each case. Several of the studies[22,23,26-28] that focused only on a limited number of specific conditions were able to use panels of clinicians to define severity for those conditions and for relevant comorbidities. Some of these investigators adopted various instruments for severity measurement, such as APACHE II, Disease Staging, and the Physiologic Stability Index Score (see table 1). However, some of these studies[23,25,28] used rather simplistic measures of complexity, such as the existence of any secondary diagnosis or the number of other diagnoses. This is an insensitive way to measure complexity, because secondary diagnoses can range from minor conditions that do not increase the risk of death at all to major problems, such as cardiac arrests. Also, it seems likely that the riskiness of various secondary diagnoses will vary depending on the primary diagnosis.

Certain interactions are undoubtedly more dangerous than others. Ideally, condition-specific risk factors should be used. Moreover, the studies that define a risk factor simply as the presence of any secondary diagnosis included iatrogenic events as patient risk factors. This was clearly not intended, because the purpose was to measure the patient's risk factors at the time of admission, not to confound risk factors with hospital performance. Although it is not always possible to separate preexisting comorbidity from complications that occurred during the hospital stay, some attempt should be made to exclude the more obvious complications (e.g., postoperative wound infections and foreign object left in surgical wound) when these conditions appear as secondary diagnoses.

In order to measure the effect of provider performance on patient outcomes, we must control for all of the factors that may affect patient outcomes to the extent that it is possible to do so. Given our existing data sets and measurement tools, it is clearly not possible to control for all of these other factors, especially those risk factors related to the patient's social condition or health behavior. It is possible, however, to use the information contained in existing databases to develop some reasonable proxies for some of the risk factors, other than provider performance, related to patient outcomes. One can use the information readily available in hospital discharge abstract data to assess the risk of various adverse outcomes associated with patients' diagnoses (principal and secondary), ages, and surgical procedures. Once we control for these risk factors, we can obtain much better (although not perfect) comparisons of hospital performance.[20,29,30]

## Risk-Adjustment
It is essential to use risk-adjusted measures for outcome variables that allow valid comparisons across hospitals. The following steps must be followed:

1. In order to ensure consistency in the analysis of risk-adjusted data, it is essential to do a preliminary assessment of data quality, including coding rules, compliance with coding rules, editing for errors, inconsistencies, and uniform rules for exclusions.

2. Collect data.

3. Using the risk-adjustment models, assign the predicted probability of each relevant adverse event to each case.

4. Develop reports for each hospital, comparing predicted frequencies for each category of adverse event to the observed frequencies.

5. As part of these reports, perform statistical tests on the differences between predicted and observed frequencies to determine whether the differences are statistically significant or merely represent random variations.

6. Using these reports, develop systems profiles, comparing hospitals within the system using the multiple risk-adjusted measures.

We can use these profiles for a "first cut." Hospitals with unusual (significant) patterns of adverse occurrences should examine records and perform peer reviews to determine whether there are problems with the process of care and whether administrative actions may be required at a systems level.

Several kinds of things *should not* be done with outcome measures:

■ Do not try to rank hospitals as "good" or "bad" simply on the basis of the scores on these indices. Recognize the limitations of these measures, which are derived from discharge abstract/billing data. Relevant in-depth clinical information may be missing. We cannot always determine time sequences, i.e., did pneumonia or a UTI develop when the patient was in the hospital, or was the infection already present at the time of admission. We cannot take into account patient compliance, an obvious factor for predicting readmissions.

■ Do not assume that data quality is good, or uniform across hospitals. Problems with data quality will definitely affect hospital scores on these measures. Poor coding of comorbidities will make a hospital look worse; good coding of complications will make a hospital look worse.

■ Do not assume that a hospital that does well on one measure is necessarily doing well on the other measures. There is no evidence that this is true.

### Aggregation of Different Measures of Adverse Events

A valid index of hospital performance must encompass the multiple aspects of hospital care. It may not be possible, either conceptually or technically, to construct one all-inclusive index of the quality of hospital care. It is, however, possible to construct several indexes that validly measure important aspects of quality and then to examine the relationships among the various measures to see if they are correlated. If the various indicators are highly correlated, we eventually may be able to construct an overall (unidimensional) quality measure. If they are not correlated, we could conclude that the various components measure distinct dimensions of quality and that the separate measures are all necessary in obtaining a valid impression of a hospital's performance.

A recent analysis by DesHarnais et al.[30] analyzed the relationships among three measures that seem to be "intrinsically valid," in that they clearly are outcomes to be avoided. The three indicators—mortality, unscheduled readmissions, and complications—were adjusted for some of the clinical factors that are predictive of the occurrence of deaths, readmissions, and complications. Risk factors were established empirically within each disease category for each index. We demonstrated that hospitals' rankings on the three indexes were not correlated. This result provides some evidence that these different indexes appear to be measuring different dimensions of hospital performance. Thus, the three indexes should not be combined into a unidimensional measure of quality, at least not at the hospital level of analysis. Neither should any one measure be used to represent all three aspects of quality.

One cannot simply choose one hospitalwide measure, such as a "death rate," to validly represent a hospital's performance. Neither can one simply add up occurrences of different types of adverse events and then claim to have a unidimensional measure of hospital performance. Those hospitals that rank well in terms of mortality rates do not necessarily do well on the other measures and may have excessive readmissions or complications.

Can these different types of adverse events be weighted in a meaningful way, so that they can be combined and used as a tool to rank hospitals? Probably not. Even after careful risk adjustments and data quality control, one is still left with the problem of how to weight a death in importance, relative to a return surgery or an unscheduled readmission. Clearly they are not of the same importance, and it would not make sense to treat them as if they were.

## Institutional Responses

Given that the management of an academic health center understands the history and politics of quality of health care, has an appropriate conceptual model of quality, and develops suitable risk-adjusted quality measures, what does it then do about quality? The first step is to make sure that they share a quality strategy. The second step is to see that the strategy is implemented consistently across the three major programs of the institution—research, education, and community service (primarily care delivery).

Linder[31] suggests that there are three basic strategies that institutions can adopt on quality of care, specifically outcomes measurement. No one is against quality by definition and no one is about to argue for unreasonable prices. Therefore, all three favor cost control and quality. She describes them as:

- **Status quo organizations**—tend to target reasonable quality at a reasonable price. They tend to have medical staff as the dominant group, with individual physicians left to provide quality leadership. Outcomes information in these organizations centers on routine compliance-oriented data prepared by medical librarians and nurses.

- **Administrative control organizations**—tend to target reasonable quality at an excellent (high) price. Administration takes predominant responsibility for quality and focuses on outliers of quality and resource utilization (cost). Nurses constitute the QA staff, and reports focus on identifying outliers.

- **Professional network organizations**—tend to target for excellent quality at a reasonable price. These organizations tend to have strong medical leadership, with a joint partnership with the administrative leadership to provide excellent service. The emphasis is on ad hoc studies to inform consensus conferences using the skills of both clinical researchers and information analysts.

About the latter group, Linder writes: "Twenty percent of the hospitals had begun to take a very different approach. The administrative and medical staffs joined forces to form an organization that held quality as its first purpose. In contrast to

Model 2 (Administrative Control), they believed that financial success would follow from medical effectiveness. Their intent was not to manage the external image of quality, but to continuously assess and improve the organization's actual quality. They believed that the way to achieve this goal was through the free and open discussion of medical effectiveness among professionals. In other words, they used an informed, professional peer network, rather than an authority structure, to manage the organization's performance. The network included administrators, nurses, and physicians, and it addressed both financial and clinical issues.[31]

It would be foolish to attempt to try to classify an entire academic health center into any one of those three categories. That is one of the handicaps of academic health centers in attempting to adapt to environmental pressures. They are loosely coupled organizations that seldom respond as a whole, but rather piece by piece.[32] One department or even a division of a department might be in the status quo stage, while another is in the professional network stage. At the same time, one teaching hospital might be in the administrative control stage and other working toward professional networking.

We believe that an academic health center is best served by moving toward the professional networking approach as rapidly as its leadership can take it there. The administrative control approach would not be acceptable to the faculty over time. It does not fit with the faculty's concepts of professional autonomy or governance or leadership. Sooner or later, it will lead to a revolution on the part of the staff. The status quo approach, however, appears to set the institution's sights too low for long-run survival at worst and to be "subject to unpleasant regulatory mandates"[31] at best. That will take real medical leadership. There are leaders in academic medicine who argue that the status quo is the prevailing set of norms in academic medicine.[33]

One fear often expressed by members of the medical profession is that we are developing protocol-oriented medical automation, or "cookbook medicine." Reed warns that, "As bureaucratic protocols based on cost containment seek to homogenize heterogeneous conditions and events, and the organizational penalties for being wrong or not conforming to the uniformity in the system multiply, there will be a devaluation of concepts such as initiative, innovation, or the utilization of experientially based clinical hunches."[34]

Physicians need to adapt to the changed environment in several ways:

■ They need to overcome some of the resistance to accountability to nonphysicians (administrators, government, consumers) to form working alliances with these powerful groups.

■ To cooperate, they need to develop the behavioral skills required to function in interdisciplinary teams.

■ They need to develop a reasonable degree of sophistication with the methods and tools used to assess/measure quality and a critical appreciation of their strengths and weaknesses.

If these changes occur, it is even possible that there can be an empowerment to physicians to actively participate with others in improving the quality of care.[35] There can be a change in role and function, but potentially a gain in the ability of physicians to work with others to produce better results. Reed[34] points out that the alternatives are either a situation where professionalism inevitably disappears, as our society follows its course of economic and organizational evolution, or a situation where "physicians can be much less the prisoners of history." Physicians can choose to "either act creatively, quickly, and decisively in the interests of their profession and their society, or to acquiesce to changes planned by others."[34]

Academic health centers need to take the leadership in quality outcomes throughout each leg of the three-legged stool—research, teaching, and service (including care delivery), as well as in the institutional postures cited above.

## Research
In their capacities as contract research establishments, medical schools are among those doing most of the research on quality in health care. HCFA, NIH, and other health agencies understand that the way to get studies done is to fund them. The already extensive capacity to do clinical trials of new technology can be turned toward both prospective and retrospective studies of the older technologies that account for most of the cost of care. There is also a core of expertise to participate actively in the development of national and specialty guidelines.

### National Guidelines and Standards
At present, the two loci for studies of practice guidelines are:

■ The government, through the Agency for Health Care Policy and Research (AHCPR) and its Forum for Quality and Effectiveness in Health Care.

■ Medical specialty organizations.

One might well ask why academic health centers are not taking the lead in this process. Another might argue that they are, because the specialty groups setting practice guidelines, such as the American Society of Anesthesiologists, the American College of Physicians/American Heart Association Task Force, and the American College of Obstetrics and Gynecology, include many academics.[36] Academic health centers are also the loci of the AHCPR studies. However, the government's grants and contracts system emphasizes individual investigators. Institutional leadership does not seem to be providing medical leadership in many of these situations.

### PORT Studies
Among key AHCPR activities have been some 11 studies by Patient Outcomes Research Teams (PORT), which use administrative data bases, epidemiological methods, and outcome evaluations by patients to look at the relative effectiveness of alternative ways of diagnosing and treating high-volume conditions, including low back pain, stroke, benign prostatic hyperplasia, bed sores, urinary incontinence in adults, and depression. Medical school researchers play major roles in these large retrospective studies. Presumably, their results will be used as inputs into local consensus-building approaches and effective practice guidelines.

### Consensus Conferences
Consensus conferences would seem to be the most natural of activities for academic health centers to conduct. When called together by NIH or other agencies, the

renowned medical specialists from many medical centers gather and freely offer their opinions on the assigned subject. It would seem that most decisions at an academic health center would come about through internal consensus conferences. Yet that seldom happens. There seem to be a number of factors involved:

■ There is an honor in being asked to a national conference, with its recognition as a noted expert as well as opportunities to network with international "peers."

■ The local consensus conference would imply constraints on future behavior in a way that an extra-institutional consensus would not.

■ There is no central authority to enforce a consensus in an academic health center, and the faculty would just as soon maintain its autonomy. Maintaining professional autonomy is a key issue in the implementation of quality programs.[37]

A precursor to consensus conferences is development of process analyses within the organization that can lead to practice guidelines and standards. A good working description of practice guidelines is "Standardized specifications for care developed by a formal process that incorporates the best scientific evidence of effectiveness with expert opinion."[36]

We believe that one of the places where the leadership of AHCs should be active is in encouraging local consensus conference as an important collegial activity carrying credit both in research and in teaching.

### Epidemiological/Small Area Studies

The Minnesota experience indicates that epidemiological studies based on small-area data can also be the basis of research on quality. This can be done by individual investigators or by organized medicine in a geographic area.[6,38,39] The latter raises an interesting issue, pointing out that academic studies may be interesting but may not be generalizable to the rest of the medical community. Leape[36] outlines a number of methodological criteria that should be applied to these retrospective studies that start with automated insurance records.

These small area studies do not have to deal only with methods of treatment (technical management). These approaches should also be applied to issues of accessibility, interpersonal process, and continuity. For example, Hand et al.[40] report that the degree of compliance to technical standards (omission of hormone receptor tests and radiation therapy) varies by hospitals and drops with urban location and a higher proportion of poorly insured patients. Likewise, Lazovich et al.[41] report that breast-conserving surgery among women with Stage I and Stage II breast cancer increases with education and income.

### TQM/CQI

The quality assurance activities of the academic health center can adopt a number of strategies, as Linder has observed.[31] One of them involves adopting a research or continuous improvement attitude rather than a compliance one. It often starts with the collection and comparison of clinical indicators, even though they deal with disease and provide little information on the processes producing the results reported. However, as Marder[42] argues, "indicators and practice guidelines have a symbiotic relationship. Each adds value to the other, and their development is best performed simultaneously, rather than sequentially. The result is a continuing cycle of measurement and analysis leading to the knowledge necessary to develop the tools for quality management in health care needed in the 1990s." Work at Latter Day Saints Hospital by faculty of the University of Utah medical school indicates great promise for the combination of carefully designed treatment protocols and computer-based expert systems in complex ICU cases where the number of variables to be manipulated is beyond individuals' limited information processing capabilities.[43]

## Teaching

A symposium announcement associated with the 13th Annual Conference of the Association of American Medical Colleges (November 12-13, 1991) stated that, "The state of development of quality improvement in medical education at the present time can be characterized as embryonic. There is much to be done in the area of theory development and application. In addition, as educational institutions, medical schools have a responsibility to educate future physicians about continuous quality improvement."[44] The proposers of the symposium mention work at Harvard on continuous improvement applied to curriculum development and the Cleveland Asthma project at Case Western Reserve. Their assessment appears to be correct. Interest in continuous quality improvement as a model seems to be centered much more in hospital administrations than in medical school teaching, possibly because hospitals, under DRGs, have felt the impact of rising costs much more than faculty practice plans have. Furthermore, faculties are much more likely to acknowledge excellence in research and excellence in teaching than excellence in clinical care.[45]

Myers and Gleicher[46] report a successful intervention at Mt. Sinai Hospital in Chicago that reduced cesarian section rates by a third. A wide variety of methods were used to modify physician practice patterns, including an information system to monitor practice patterns, issuance of practice guidelines, circulation of comparisons with other institutions, peer review, and annual performance evaluations. The departmental leadership was willing to go as far as limiting privileges, if that had proved necessary.

### Practice Management

However, practice plans under RBRVS are more likely to get involved in the future in issues of cost and quality[47] if they are going to be able to fulfill their financial commitments to faculties. Initial efforts will be improved outpatient care facilities to attract patients, participation in HMOs and PPOs, running satellite centers, and more aggressive marketing of services. With that, however, will have to come concerns about customer-oriented quality of care measures. This is not likely to happen rapidly, given the current emphasis on selecting faculty practice plan executives based on their ability to do accounting, billing, and collections. They will get to the quality of care issues only when the dean or medical director becomes very active in practice management.

A likely reason for a teaching group to become involved in practice standards is utilization of a quality improvement program in a competing HMO. Gottlieb et al.[48] report the development of a number of algorithms for use by the Harvard Community Health Program (HCHP) staff and their incorporation into continuing medical education programs and into information gathering systems. They suggest that the criteria for developing algorithms are:

- Frequency, involving commonly seen clinical conditions.
- Unexplained variability in clinical practice, or resource utilization, or referral patterns.
- Conflict with internal resource constraints.
- Apparent risk management problems.
- Perceived quality of care issues with patients, clinicians, or managers.
- Introduction of new technology.
- Uncertainty about use or about cost implications.

These appear to be the criteria that would make an issue of interest to the faculty of a medical school as well. Yet it seems to be an HMO that is leading the way, presumably because the expectations of autonomy in practice activity are much less strong in a staff-model HMO such as HCHP.

Competitive stimuli, however, can force medical school staff into quality studies. For example, the faculty of an academic family medicine department became truly interested in continuity of care only when the largest employer in the community threatened to cancel its worker's compensation/industrial medicine contract with the department because of visit and waiting time costs related to lack of physician continuity. There had been many complaints about continuity of care from individual patients, but the staff became involved only when threatened with the loss of this major account. Most of the time, lost patients disappeared one at a time without a ripple.

Because of the insulation of academic departments from such information through the hospital and the practice plan, improvements in care are most likely to come about when the faculty decides that the learners in the institution must learn to practice the right way. Quality will most likely come about when the faculty decides that students (undergraduate and residents) must see exemplary practice in action. It will take medical leadership within the faculty to make that an organizational objective. In doing so, the leadership must also deal with the fact that faculty in a teaching setting are significantly less efficient than their competitors who are not teaching. As Garg et al. point out, this means facing up to some of the true cost of teaching in the clinical setting, especially the increasingly important outpatient clinic.[49]

### Inclusion in Curriculum Development

Headrick et al.[35] report on the four-year educational project at Case Western Reserve University School of Medicine to introduce continuous quality improvement into the curriculum. It is part of an eight-week clerkship at one of a number of urban and suburban clinic sites. The application was highly constrained by time, multiple sites, and poor cost and patient information systems. The assignment given each student focused on outcomes of both costs and symptoms and then on process improvement. The strength of the reported barriers to these future physicians' learning about costs at all was amazing. The students did seem to get somewhere with cost-gathering and with process improvement, but the curriculum still lacked the skills development necessary to work well in or to lead group processes, critical skills if the knowledge gained is to be applied elsewhere.

The authors report that the Cleveland Asthma Project is one of its kind. "Yet it is still rudimentary in terms of what physicians need to be leaders in process improvement. Yet the degree to which hospitals, business leaders, and doctors are committed to CQI or TQM sends a signal to medical students about how important such efforts are. If students, residents, and physicians find indifference all around them about costs, outcome, and process of care, they will promptly forget what was taught....The project has made us realize that good care must be provided in partnership between providers, payers, and patients. That parts of the process lie beyond the physician's office or emergency room should have come as no surprise, but we have failed to act on this knowledge. With a close ongoing partnership, perhaps we can do so in the future."[55]

We owe a debt of gratitude to the CWRU team for making this start, but it is damning of academic medicine that this is the current state-of-the-art in continuous improvement. As the above quote indicates, the concepts of quality, with or without continuous improvement, are going to permeate medical practice only when they permeate the medical school and its teaching settings.

### Cost Consciousness

Control of costs can be taught both directly and indirectly. For example, Durand et al.[50] report that third-year medical students who are able to organize hypotheses about patients' problems best are more likely to order the appropriate diagnostic tests. The ordering of necessary tests is not affected by this factor, but the ordering of inappropriate tests is. There is, however, much more to be studied about the correlates of lower cost behaviors.

For example, Feinglass et al.[51] report that costs go down significantly in teaching settings as autonomy in medical decision-making allowed by attending physicians goes up. The authors suggest that this reflects the busy residents' inherently conservative practice style that favors moving patients out. One might also interpret it as reflecting defensive medicine directed against nit-picking attendings. At least it indicates the variability introduced into the treatment system by lack of commonly accepted treatment processes (protocols) even within specific teaching institutions.

### Multilevel and Multidisciplinary Teams

As the Cleveland Asthma Project indicates, the medical education environment has significant problems in finding ways to give medical students and residents theoretical and experiential tools to work in multilevel and multidisciplinary teams that are necessary to improve the process of patient care. One of the reported findings of that study was the insight that the process of care is much more complex than the medical teachers had assumed and that an effective outcome depends on factors outside the clinic setting as well as inside it.[55] Hellman[52] notes similar problems within the university in terms of bringing to bear the many relevant disciplines of the university on modern health care problems. He argues, "Despite this impressive panoply of opportunities for better health care, the system has disturbing maldistribution, with little organized preventive medicine. All these changes have vexing ethical and social policy considerations. At such times there are unique opportunities for scholarly thought and discussion involving much of the university, with the possibility that changes may be directed by such considerations."

## Service

Academic health centers are the institutions that set the standard for health care quality. There are real questions about the quality of that care. A major study indicates that 3-4 percent of hospital admissions suffered adverse events due to negligence or medical mismanagement.[53,54] This study does not report the error rates for teaching institutions separately, but even if they are lower than anticipated, they still indicate that there is great room for improvement in the technical quality of health care. When one adds in the negative experiences of the customer while being served and when billed, there is much work to be done.[35]

### Practice Model Assumptions

Perhaps the most important impact of the delivery of service in academic health centers is the model of practice that it develops in the minds of its learners. Many physicians tend to stick with what they learned during that period of their lives, and many values are internalized there. What are the implications of the emphasis on income generation in many teaching clinics? What is the impact of that experience on future attitudes toward process improvement? What is the learning about how variation in the treatment process is viewed and dealt with? How is process analysis to go forward in the practice setting with its ruthless time pressures? Clearly, academic health centers have to continue to wrestle with these issues.

The results may be favorable to academic health centers as well as unfavorable. Caper[4] shows that the conservative admission pattern of university/teaching hospitals may more than offset the higher technology and costs of such institutions. Johnson[36] makes a similar argument concerning quality of care. He argues that teaching institutions have something to crow about. The Office of Technology Assessment's meta-study[53] gives no indications that teaching institutions have poorer quality results than nonteaching institutions. Certainly, as Caper argues,[4] the time for stopping stonewalling and for taking the lead in quality issues is at hand.

## Organizational Responses

### Marketing/PR

As Linder points out,[31] organizations that try to influence the image of quality through public relations and marketing are likely to end up badly. The public's perception of quality depends on comparison of expected quality versus experienced quality. If one works hard to convince someone that quality is there, one is as likely to raise expectations as to bias perceptions. Therefore, if the quality is in fact not raised but the expectation of it is raised, the perception gap is being widened. Any attempt to bias that perception favorably is likely to backfire.

On the other hand, there is merit in educating the public about how to judge quality. This involves managing expectations by helping the public determine what to look for and where to find it. There is a wealth of new information being provided on outcomes that is raw data and must be interpreted. Here the public could use help. Many states are requiring the disclosure of patient care quality indicators, patient care outcomes, and medical staff qualifications. Despite hospitals' reluctance to share this information, the data will get out to the public and to the press. So will information from the National Practitioner Data Bank. Both hospitals and physicians will have to explain what this means to themselves and to their patients.[57]

| Table 2. Physician Attributes Prized by Hospitals, as Seen by Physicians and Hospitals[57] | | |
|---|---|---|
| | **% Reporting "Very Important"** | |
| **Physician Attribute** | **Among Hospital CEOs** | **Among MDs** |
| Clinical quality/technical competence | 97% | 93% |
| Relationship with patients/reputation | 94% | 94% |
| Cost-effectiveness in hospital practice | 92% | 78% |

## Mission statement

Many hospitals have clear statements of the importance of quality in their mission statements. Some go further in seeing to it that all employees are aware of the quality content of that mission statement and can communicate it when asked to do so. Even with these broad statements, there are differences as to operational meanings. For example, the Arthur Andersen study shows that there is still a difference of opinion about the relative importance of cost effectiveness between hospitals and physicians. The physician attributes most valued by hospitals, as seen by hospitals and by physicians are shown in table 2, above. After the listed attributes, the percentages fall off. Note that by far the greatest disagreement between the hospital CEOs and physicians is over the importance of cost-effectiveness.

## Outreach/Access/Population Base

Lewis and Sheps argue that academic health centers should take responsibility for a specific population base so that issues such as prevention and access are addressed.[58] As care moves in the direction of capitation payments, most academic health centers will be faced with such a choice again and again. Only then are basic issues such as prevention, perceived quality of care, and access likely to be addressed fully. Until then the faculty is likely to continue to choose autonomy over accountability.

The academic health center must have a philosophy about whether or not it will be responsible for a population base above and beyond that sporadically attracted by the reputation of its specialist faculty. This will center on the nature and purpose of the primary care delivered by the faculty. The academic health center must decide whether or not the primary care that it delivers is the core of its undertaking or merely an appendage. Vinten-Johansen and Riska[59] characterize the choices here and the debate over them as being over how to maintain professional autonomy between Oslerians and Flexnerians. Those value systems have to be reconciled if the institution is to pull itself together to agree on quality of care in its fullest sense.

## Organization of Care

Quality is both a value and a cooperative process in an academic health center. Therefore, it must be reinforced by the governance processes of the institutions involved. Faculty do pay attention to quality in the tenure and promotion processes of the medical school. They must, however, also be intensively involved in it in the governance of the teaching hospital. Shortell[60,61] outlines the mechanisms that a hospital has for involving the physician staff in its governance processes, including many quality activities, such as the various peer review activities and the board of trustees. He also points out that this process has to be managed carefully to bring younger staff along in the skills necessary to maintain an effective governance process over time.

Even though Shortell emphasizes the need to integrate or bond physicians operating in a private-practice, fee-for-service mode that is becoming less and less prevalent, his points are still relevant to the AHC. Physicians must still be courted to make them buy into and conform to institutional norms, such as those of quality.

The introduction of cost control measures, such as DRGs, has created new motivations for quality improvement, as well as some new points of potential conflict. As care-giving organizations move toward a single package price for services such as a normal obstetrical delivery, the hospital and some physicians have a community of interest in having a safe and an efficient process that attracts and satisfies patients. If obstetricians are losing business because the care is traditional, not attractive, and costly, the hospital and the obstetricians can cooperate to come up with a competitive process. But there can be other situations, such as the interaction between radiologists and the hospital administration, where the motivations of fee-for-service physician payment and DRGs put the two in an adversarial position on cost and perhaps on quality of care.

In the managed care setting, there is less apparent conflict between management and the caregivers than in a fee-for-service setting. However, pressures for productivity and reduced costs can still lead to conflict between the two. Somehow, the governance process has to allow these issues to be brought to light, discussed, and settled if the organization is to maintain any momentum in the quality area. There are also possible conflicts within the roles of the care givers. On one hand, the primary care giver is expected to be an advocate and facilitator for the patient. On the other hand, the primary physician is expected to control costs by being a gatekeeper to specialists and an auditor of their performance. The governance process must address these issues squarely if the patient and the physician are to feel comfortable with the process.

Still another area where the governance process must elicit physician cooperation and involvement is in the area of continuous quality improvement and quality assurance. Many physicians see quality assurance as an intrusion by nonphysicians. Quality improvement programs, if they involve the physicians early, offer a chance to regain some of that perceived loss of autonomy as well as opportunities for massive process improvements.

### Legal Screen of Peer Review
Most states have laws that shield quality assurance studies done on behalf of the institution's board of trustees from discovery proceedings in malpractice cases. Some laws are being amended to cover CQI program data as well under the same principles of law. The legal status of practice guidelines and their use is less clear. "Although it is possible that such policies and guidelines could be admitted into evidence to show that a provider breached a legal duty or standard of care owed a patient, it is uncertain whether these risk-control standards could ultimately pass the evidentiary rules of relevancy or materiality in a given law suit."[62] Borbas et al.[39] also cite the use of the argument in Minnesota that solid data are more effective for defending physicians' practices than expert witnesses."

While many observers express concern about the use of continuous quality management in discovery proceedings associated with malpractice suits, Holzer[62] suggests that it is more likely that "the consensus-based process of creating clinical standards and guidelines specifically for controlling professional liability losses is itself a powerful and emerging standard for health care risk management programs." This would be especially important should the initial data be borne out that the quality of health care is generally enhanced by the use of health care protocols *per se*.[45]

### Authority Patterns

McLaughlin and Kaluzny[37] emphasize the autonomy and authority barriers that must be overcome in introducing quality concepts into clinical practice. The debate between Berwick and Zusman[63-65] shows two contrasting points of view. Berwick emphasizes the TQM approach, with its multidisciplinary emphasis, arguing that clinical care is "a network of deep interdependencies involving other professionals, nonprofessional staff, information systems, policies and procedures, physical systems, and other influences on their own work and on the patients they serve. Sometimes physicians indeed act alone. But usually not." Zusman argues that quality assurance is a well-developed, stable approach that deals adequately with clinical quality but should "not consider cost of care a quality issue," that cost is a utilization management staff responsibility. In his ideal hospital, administration "leaves monitoring of the quality of professional care to the QA system (or more strictly, leaves to the QA system that care that falls under the medical staff privileging system) while it monitors the quality of all other services and products that the hospital either purchases or produces."

The current structuring of medical schools and teaching hospitals supports the "traditional" system outlined by Zusman. Yet the results seem to leave much to be desired from a clinical, cost, and patient perspective. It is time for the management of the academic health center to take a strong position in this conflictful arena.

## Conclusions

Quality is something that all physicians favor, including faculties and residents. It is not, as many would like to believe, something that happens without planning and conscientious effort. The outside world is demanding of academic health centers, as well as their competition, the highest quality at a reasonable price. Information with which to make assessments of outcome performance in health care is becoming widely available. The academic health center can fight to maintain professional autonomy by pushing the lay assessors back, or it can take the lead by becoming expert on quality assessment and applying those skills to its ongoing operations. It can then educate the public in how to interpret the impact of age, comorbidity, and other factors on outcomes measures. It can include the measures developed in its research into its teaching and into its delivery of care. It can educate its learners in how to participate in the processes of quality improvement, to cooperate with other disciplines and professional groups, to lead the way in analysis and process design, and to help develop consensus about what is currently known and what warrants further study. It can go much further in empowering all its constituents to follow the scientific method at a pragmatic level in all aspects of medicine and in all settings to the benefit of its consumers. It can move from being on the defensive about consumer-oriented quality and how it is measured toward being its primary advocate.

# References

1.  Graham, N. *Quality Assurance in Hospitals.* Rockville, Md.: Aspen Publishers, 1990, p. 6-7.

2.  McAninch, M. "Accrediting Agencies and the Search for Quality in Health Care." In *Handbook of Quality Assurance in Mental Health,* edited by Stricker, G., and Rodriguez, A. New York, N.Y.: Plenum Press, 1988.

3.  Starr, P. *The Social Transformation of American Medicine.* New York, N.Y.: Basic Books, Inc., 1982.

4.  Caper, P. "Defining Quality in Medical Care." *Health Affairs* 7(1):49-61, Spring, 1988.

5.  Donabedian, A. *The Criteria and Standards of Quality.* Ann Arbor, Mich.: Health Administration Press, 1982.

6.  Wennberg, J., and Gittelson, A. "Small Area Variations in Health Care Delivery." *Science* 82(4117):1102-8, Dec. 14, 1973.

7.  Paul-Shaheen, P., and others. "Small Area Analysis: A Review of the North American Literature." *Journal of Health Politics, Policy, and Law* 12(4):741-809, Winter 1987.

8.  Leape, L. "Unnecessary Surgery." *Health Services Research* 24(3):351-407, Aug. 1987.

9.  Adams, D., and others. "The Complications of Coronary Arteriography." *Circulation* 48(3):609-18, Sept. 1973.

10. Brook, R., and others. *A Review of the Literature on Cholecystectomy: Findings, Complications, Utilization Rates, Costs, Efficacy, and Indications.* Santa Monica, Calif.: RAND Corp., 1975.

11. Roos, L., and others. "Using Computers to Identify Complications after Surgery." *American Journal of Public Health* 75(11):1288-95, Nov. 1985.

12. Chassin, M. "Quality of Care: Time to Act." *JAMA* 226(24):3472-3, Dec. 25, 1991.

13. U.S. Congress, Office of Technology Assessment. *The Quality of Medical Care: Information for Consumers,* OTA-H-386. Washington, D.C.: U.S. Government Printing Office, June 1988.

14. Donabedian, A. "Criteria and Standards for Quality Assessment and Monitoring." *Quality Review Bulletin* 14(3):99-108, March 1986.

15. Donabedian, A. *Explorations in Quality Assessment and Monitoring,* Vol. 1. Ann Arbor, Mich.: Health Administration Press, 1980, pp. 95-7.

16. Moses, L., and Mosterrer, F. "Institutional Differences in Postoperative Death Rates: Commentary on Some of the Findings of the National Halothane Study." *JAMA* 203(7):492-4, Feb. 12, 1968.

17. Wagner, D., and others. "The Case for Adjusting Hospital Death Rates for Severity of Illness." *Health Affairs* 5(2):148-53, Summer 1986.

18. Pollack, M., and others. "Accurate Prediction of the Outcome of Pediatric Intensive Care: A New Quantitative Method." *New England Journal of Medicine* 316(3):134-9, Jan. 15, 1987.

19. Knaus, W., and others. "An Evaluation of Outcome from Intensive Care in Major Medical Centers." *Annals of Internal Medicine* 104(3):410-8, March 1986.

20. DesHarnais, S., and others. "The Risk-Adjusted Mortality Index: A New Measure of Hospital Performance." *Medical Care* 26(12):1129-48, Dec. 1988.

21. Roemer, M., and others. "A Proposed Hospital Quality Index: Hospital Death Rates Adjusted for Case Severity." *Health Services Research* 3(2):96-118, Summer 1968.

22. Flood, A., and others. "Effectiveness in Professional Organizations: The Impact of Surgeons and Surgical Staff Organizations on the Quality of Care in Hospitals." *Health Services Research* 17(4):341-66, Winter 1982.

23. Luft, H., and Hunt, S. "Evaluating Individual Hospital Quality through Outcome Statistics." *JAMA* 255(20):2780-4, May 23-30, 1986.

24. Blumberg, M. "Risk-Adjusting Health Care Outcomes: A Methodological Review." *Medical Care Review* 43(2):351-93, Fall 1986.

25. Hebel, J., and others. "Assessment of Hospital Performance by Use of Death Rates: A Recent Case History." *JAMA* 248(23):3131-5, Dec. 17, 1982.

26. Sloan, F., and others. "In-Hospital Mortality of Surgical Patients: Is there an Empirical Basis for Standard Setting?" *Surgery* 99(4):446-54, April 1986.

27. Wennberg, J., and others. "Use of Claims Data Systems to Evaluate Health Care Outcomes: Mortality and Reoperation Following Prostatectomy." *JAMA* 257(7):933-6, Feb. 20, 1987.

28. Kelly, J., and Hellinger, F. "Physician and Hospital Factors Associated with Mortality of Surgical Patients." *Medical Care* 24(9):785-800, Sept. 1986.

29. DesHarnais, S., and others. "Measuring Hospital Performance: The Development and Validation of Risk-Adjusted Indexes of Mortality, Readmissions, and Complications." *Medical Care* 28(12):1127-41, Dec. 1990.

30. DesHarnais, S., and others. "Measuring Outcomes of Hospital Care Using Multiple Risk-Adjusted Indexes." *Health Services Research* 26(4):425-45, Oct. 1991.

31. Linder, J. "Outcomes Measurement: Compliance Tool or Strategic Initiative?" *Health Care Management Review* 16(4):21-33, Fall 1991.

32. Weick, K. "Educational Organizations as Loosely Coupled Systems." *Administrative Science Quarterly* 21(3):1-19, March 1976.

33. Cotton, P. "Medical Schools Receive a Message: Reform Yourselves, Then Take on Health Care System." *JAMA* 266(20):2802-4, Nov. 27, 1991.

34. Reed, R., and Evans, D. "The Deprofessionalization of Medicine: Causes, Effects, and Responses.", *JAMA* 258(22):3279-82, Dec. 11, 1987.

35. Headrick, L., and others. "Introducing Quality Improvement Thinking to Medical Students: The Cleveland Asthma Project." *Quality Review Bulletin* 17(8):254-60, Aug, 1991.

36. Leape, L. "Practice Guidelines and Standards: An Overview." *Quality Review Bulletin* 16(2):42-9, Feb. 1990.

37. McLaughlin, C., and Kaluzny, A. "Total Quality Management in Health: Making it Work." *Health Care Management Review* 15(3):7-14, Summer 1990.

38. Chassin, M., and others. "Variations in the Use of Medical and Surgical Services by the Medicare Population." *New England Journal of Medicine* 314(5):285-90, Jan. 30, 1986.

39. Borbas, C., and others. "The Minnesota Clinical Comparison and Assessment Project." *Quality Review Bulletin* 16(2):87-92, Feb. 1990.

40. Hand, R., and others. "Hospital Variables Associated with Quality of Care for Breast Cancer Patients." *JAMA* 266(24):3429-32, Dec. 25, 1991.

41. Lazovich, D., and others. "Underutilization of Breast-Conserving Surgery and Radiation Therapy Among Women with Stage I and II Breast Cancer." *JAMA* 266(24):3433-8, Dec. 25, 1991.

42. Marder, R. "Relationship of Clinical Indicators and Practice Guidelines." *Quality Review Bulletin* 16(2):60, Feb. 1990.

43. Morris, A. "Protocols, ECCO2R, and the Evaluation of New ARDS Therapy." *Japanese Journal of Intensive Care Medicine* 16:61-3, 1992.

44. "Continuous Quality Improvement in Medical Education: Applying Industrial Models to Medical Education." *Academic Medicine* 66(9, Suppl.):S86, Sept. 1991.

45. Bentley, J., and others. "Faculty Practice Plans: The Organization and Characteristics of Academic Medical Practice." *Academic Medicine* 66(8):433-9, Aug. 1991.

46. Myers, S., and Gleicher, N. "A Successful Program to Reduce Cesarean Section Rates: Friendly Persuasion." *Quality Review Bulletin* 17(5):162-6, May 1991.

47. Hillman, A., and others. "An Academic Medical Center's Experience with Mandatory Managed Care for Medicaid Recipients." *Academic Medicine* 66(3):134-8, March 1991.

48. Gottlieb, L., and others. "Clinical Practice Guidelines in an HMO: Development and Implementation in a Quality Improvement Model." *Quality Review Bulletin* 16(2):81, Feb. 1990.

49. Garg, M., and others. "Primary Care Teaching Physicians' Losses of Productivity and Revenue at Three Ambulatory Care Centers." *Academic Medicine* 66(6):348-53, June 1991.

50. Durand, R., and others. "Association Between Third-year Medical Students' Abilities to Organize Hypotheses about Patients' Problems and to Order Appropriate Diagnostic Tests." *Academic Medicine* 66(11):702-4, Nov. 1991.

51. Feinglass, J., and others. "The Relationship of Residents' Autonomy and Use of a Teaching Hospital's Resources." *Academic Medicine* 66(9):549-52, Sept. 1991.

52. Hellman, S. "The Intellectual Quarantine of American Medicine," *Academic Medicine* 66(5):245-8, May 1991.

53. Brennan, T., and others. "Incidence of Adverse Events and Negligence in Hospitalized Patients." *New England Journal of Medicine* 324(6):370-6, Feb. 6, 1991.

54. Leape, L., and others. "The Nature of Adverse Events in Hospitalized Patients." *New England Journal of Medicine* 324(6):377-84, Feb. 6, 1991.

55. Sahney, V., and Warden, G. "The Quest for Quality and Productivity in Health Services." *Frontiers of Health Services Management* 7(4):2-40, Summer 1991.

56. Johnson, D. "HCFA's Mortality Statistics Boost Teaching Hospitals." *Health Care Strategic Management* 8(1):2-3, Jan. 1990.

57. Arthur Anderson and the American College of Healthcare Executives. *The Future of Medical Care: Physician and Hospital Relationships.* Chicago, Ill.: American College of Healthcare Executives, 1991.

58. Lewis, I., and Sheps, C. *The Sick Citadel: The American Academic Medical Center and the Public Interest.* Cambridge, Mass.: Oelgeschlager, Gunn and Hain, 1983.

59. Vinten-Johansen, P., and Riska, E. "New Oslerians and Real Flexnerians: The Response to Threatened Professional Autonomy." *International Journal of Health Services* 21(1):75-108, 1991.

60. Shortell, S. "The Medical Staff of the Future: Replanting the Garden." *Frontiers of Health Services Management* 1(3):3-48, Feb. 1985.

61. Shortell, S. "Revisiting the Garden: Medicine and Management in the 1990s." *Frontiers of Health Services Management* 7(1):3-32, Fall 1990.

62. Holzer, J. "The Advent of Clinical Standards for Professional Liability." *Quality Review Bulletin* 16(2):72-9, Feb. 1991.

63. Berwick, D. "Peer Review and Quality Management: Are They Compatible?" *Quality Review Bulletin* 16(7):246-51, July 1990.

64. Berwick, D. "Reply: `Peer Review and Quality Management: Are They Compatible?'" *Quality Review Bulletin* 16(12):419-20, Dec. 1990.

65. Zusman, J. "Letter: 'Peer Review and Quality Management: Are They Compatible?'" *Quality Review Bulletin* 16(12):418-9, Dec. 1991.

*Susan I. DesHarnais, PhD, is Associate Professor, School of Public Health, and Curtis P. McLaughlin, DBA, is Professor of Business Administration, Kenan-Flagler Business School, University of North Carolina, Chapel Hill, N.C.*

# Chapter 9

# Legislation and the Academic Health Center

*by Lois Margaret Nora, MD, JD,*
*and Brett Eric Reetz, JD*

**A**cademic Health Centers (AHCs) are relied upon to further national goals of improved health and health services. An analysis of existing legislation reveals an apparent congressional mandate for the existence and survival of AHCs. It also shows that national health policy relies heavily on these institutions to solve health problems and to meet goals of research, technologic innovations, and expanded health services. This chapter will review some of the legislation that supports AHCs and directs their activities, as well as some of the problems of efficacy intrinsic to the legislation.

Federal legislation regarding AHCs can be dissected to reveal two major objectives. First, certain aspects of legislation specifically encourage and provide for the existence of AHCs. It is important to note that federal legislation does not expressly mandate the existence of AHCs. Encouragement of AHCs' existence usually occurs through providing for direct funding of these institutions. Second, other aspects of legislation encourage AHCs to develop and provide solutions to a variety of health problems, ranging from specific diseases that Congress deems worthy of attention to the curing of social ills, such as the disproportionately small number of minority health care workers.

It is important to note that most legislation does not fall solely into one category or the other. Individual legislation frequently includes measures designed to support the existence of AHCs and directives that AHCs effectuate policy. These two characteristics of legislation, analyzed together, make it clear that Congress finds critical the continued presence of AHCs.

Another significant purpose of the legislation is to create bodies of expertise that can advise Congress and government agencies on AHC issues. Two examples, discussed in greater detail below, are the Council on Graduate Medical Education and the Advisory Council on Education of Health Professionals. These Councils help reinforce the partnership between AHCs and the federal agency that the legislation encourages.

The bulk of legislation favorable to AHCs is found in Title 42 of the United States Code.[1] Title 42 provides comprehensive and extensive programs that aid AHCs. These programs include grants for construction, mortgage guarantees, money for program development, and faculty development opportunities, among others. More than any other body of legislation, it reveals the intentions and concerns of Congress related to AHCs.

Congressional support of AHCs begins with the actual financial support for physical plants. Congress has empowered the Secretary of the Department of Housing and Urban Development to provide financial resources for AHCs in a number of ways, including money for construction of particular facilities, technical assistance, and mortgage insurance.

The Secretary has been granted authority to provide mortgage insurance for hospitals and to provide for the guarantee of refinancing of existing mortgages of some institutions.[23] The purpose of this legislation is to assist the construction of urgently needed hospitals for the care and treatment of persons who are acutely ill or who require medical care and related services of the kind customarily furnished only (or more effectively) by hospitals.[4] Although this legislation does not specifically list AHCs as institutions to benefit from the legislation, AHCs do fall squarely within the definition of facilities provided for under the section.

Under this legislation, mortgage insurance may be provided despite other avenues of support available to the hospital. Additional security or collateral to guarantee such support cannot be required, and publicly owned or supported hospitals cannot be required to meet more stringent eligibility or other requirements. This legislation also provides for the guarantee of refinancing of existing mortgages of some institutions. Amendments to the legislation have increased the amounts available to each institution.

The Secretary is also authorized to make grants to assist in the construction of teaching facilities for the training of physicians, dentists, pharmacists, optometrists, and other health professionals.[5] Grants to construct teaching facilities may be made to schools that provide only the first two years of undergraduate medical education if this may result in the development of full-fledged schools of medicine. Monies may be granted to public and not-for-profit entities to assist in the construction of ambulatory, primary care teaching facilities for the training of physicians and dentists. The definition of facilities is quite broad; even research laboratories can qualify for the monies if it is necessary for, and appropriate to, the conduct of comprehensive ambulatory, primary care training.

Title 42 provides additional assistance to institutions receiving monies under this grant. The Secretary is empowered to provide technical assistance for the design and construction of training facilities.[6] The combination of resources can stimulate the development of these facilities.

Several purposes are served through allocation of funds in this manner. By making monies available in specific areas, national health policy goals are emphasized. Examples are the grants directed toward primary medical and dental care.[7] The programs create partnerships between AHCs and the government body, with some control over the grants retained by the federal agency. For example, the Secretary is allowed to recover the amount of the grant, plus interest, if, at any time in the subsequent 20 years from the date of the initial grant, the owner ceases to be a public or not-for-profit school.[8]

Title 42 creates several mechanisms for communication between the Secretary and persons involved in medical education and in AHCs. (The term "Secretary," when used in the context of Title 42, refers to the Secretary of Health and Human Services and any other officer or employee of the Department of Health and Human Services to whom the authority involved has been delegated.) The Advisory Council on Education for Health Professionals was established to advise the Secretary in the preparation of general regulations and with respect to policy matters arising in the administration of health research and teaching facilities and training of professional health personnel.[9] The Council consists of the Secretary (or his or her delegate) as chair and 21 additional members. Thirteen of the members are representatives of the health professions schools assisted under programs authorized under the legislation, and six members of the council are selected for their experience in university administration. Of the eight remaining members, two are health professions students.[10]

The Council make-up, and its areas of activity, reflect the reliance of Congress on the administrative and intellectual resources of AHCs in order to properly administer programs created for AHCs. This is reflected in the use of the Advisory Council in funding decisions. The construction and technical assistance grants described above are based, in part, on the input of the Council.[11] The council is dominated by persons representing the interests that will be benefitted by the funding.

The Council on Graduate Medical Education (CGME) is another committee established by Title 42 legislation.[12] The CGME has an extremely broad mandate. The committee advises several congressional committees, as well as the Secretary, on topics that include the distribution and supply of physicians in the United States, issues relating to foreign medical graduates, and the financing of programs of graduate medical education. The committee also has the charge of encouraging institutions that provide graduate medical education to voluntarily achieve recommendations of the Council.

While some legislation providing for the construction of facilities has underlying policy concerns, other legislation highlights these policy concerns to an even greater degree. Legislative efforts to promote family medicine in AHCs are an example. Grants are available to assist with the costs of projects to establish, maintain, and improve academic administrative units that provide clinical instruction in family medicine.[13] Priority is to be given to those applicants that demonstrate a commitment to family medicine in their medical education training program.[14]

Another example is legislation regarding funding directed toward the development of Area Health Education Centers.[15] A wide variety of health policy goals are mentioned in the legislation, including improved distribution and utilization of health personnel in the health delivery system, regionalization of education responsibilities of the health professional schools, and improved health care delivery, including nutrition evaluation and counseling, to previously underserved populations.[16] This highlights the expansive policy concerns that Congress seeks to address through this form of legislation. These concerns are at a local level (e.g., the previously underserved population that will now be served) and a national level (e.g., encouraging the training of primary care physicians).

A review of federal legislation highlights some of the areas of medical expertise that the government wishes to encourage. Grants are made available for the planning, development, and operation of approved residency programs that emphasize training in general internal medicine and general pediatrics.[17] Schools can get financial assistance in meeting the costs of projects to improve training in geriatric medicine.[18] These projects can expand existing instruction in this area, support faculty training, and establish new affiliations with senior centers, among other things. Preventive medicine is another area to which monies have been dedicated.[19]

Legislative support of AHCs extends beyond the construction of facilities and the development of programs geared toward providing direct care providers, however. Funding is available for the education of administrators as well. Public and not-for-profit private education entities, including social work schools but excluding accredited schools of public health, may receive grants to support graduate education programs in health administration, hospital administration, and health planning.[20] Projects designed to identify and recruit highly qualified individuals, including disadvantaged persons, into the allied health professions can be funded.

Congress also allocates money to institutions, including AHCs, that address concerns about specific disease entities. One of the most notable is funding that is being directed toward Human Immunodeficiency Virus (HIV) infection and the Acquired Immune Deficiency Syndrome (AIDS). For example, the Department of Health and Human Services provided $3.3 million in fiscal year 1989 to create the AIDS Regional Education Training Centers.[21] The program has many goals, including multidisciplinary curriculum development, support for area practitioners, assistance for patients in gaining access to research opportunities, and development of culturally relevant materials for the community served. The Centers are intended to operate in collaboration with health professional schools, community hospitals, health departments, and other organization involved in the provision of care for HIV-related conditions. AHCs provide a major resource in the delivery of this care.

Support of AHCs can be seen in rules promulgated by administrative agencies as well as the Congress. Health Care Financing Administration (HCFA) policies also support the activities of AHCs. Historically, Medicare has paid a share of the net direct and indirect costs of approved medical education activities. The regulations currently define approved educational activities to mean formally organized or planned programs of study usually engaged in by providers in order to enhance the quality of care in an institution.[22] These activities include approved training programs for physicians, nurses, and certain paramedical health professionals. Allowable costs include direct salaries and fringe benefits of resident staff, salaries related to supervision by teaching physicians, and indirect costs that are appropriately allocated to the particular medical education costs center.

The Department of Veterans Affairs is an example of a federal agency that relies upon AHCs to accomplish its goal of providing health care services. AHCs serve as advisors on health care to the Department of Veterans Affairs, and some AHC facilities and personnel act as direct care providers. The Advisory Commission on the Future Structure of Veterans Health Care was directed by the Department of Veterans Affairs in 1990 to undertake an exhaustive examination of the entire health care system.[23] The authorization specifically lists academic medicine and research as areas to draw Commission membership from. Title 38 of the United States Code allows the Secretary to enter into agreements with medical schools, hospitals, and research centers for exchange of medical information, techniques, and services.[24]

An unfortunate reality is that funding provided by Congress is frequently inadequate to effectuate the desired results. While this problem is certainly not limited to AHCs, AHCs are effected by it. Despite clear federal mandates for the existence of AHCs and for various programs, adequate resources for the desired programs are not always made available. It is paradoxical that Congress relies so heavily on the continued existence and offerings of AHCs while at the same time inadequately funding the institutions.

One example of this paradox is the cooperative agreement among the Department of Health and Human Services, the Centers for Disease Control, and the National Institute for Occupational Safety and Health to assist the nation's primary care medicine residencies in providing training to medical students and residents.[25] The purpose of this program is to enhance the education and practice of graduates of primary care programs in the field of occupational and environmental health. It is intended that this will be accomplished by linking the clinical faculty from primary care medicine residency programs with experts in occupational and environmental medicine. Specific goals that have been identified include expanding the number of primary care programs teaching occupational and environmental health, expanding the number of clinical faculty qualified to provide instruction, establishing a consultative network for patient referral, developing and implementing a model educational program to disseminate information on HIV/AIDS infection in certain health care settings, and conducting a conference to report the results of the project.

This program had funding in 1991 of $200 thousand dollars.[26] This is clearly inadequate to accomplish the identified tasks. Even though the program goals would be unattainable without AHCs, they are equally unattainable given the lack of funding.

Another example of the lack of monies to meet health policy goals is the Proposed Funding Priorities for Grants for Faculty Development in Family Medicine, as set forth by the Department of Health and Human Services.[27] This authorizes the awarding of grants to a wide variety of institutions, including AHCs, to assist in meeting the costs of planning, developing, and operating programs for the training of physicians who plan to teach in family medicine training programs. In addition, it authorizes assistance in meeting the cost of supporting physicians who are trainees in such programs and who plan to teach in family medicine training programs.

This program is merely a contingency action taken to ensure that timely awarding of grants is possible should monies become available for the program. No money was available to fund the program at the time of its drafting. The program was renewed on November 13, 1991, but, again, no funds were available.

In review of the many legislative measures promulgated by Congress and federal agencies, it is obvious that there is a congressional mandate for the existence of AHCs. It is clear that this mandate is based upon the services AHCs can provide in meeting national health policy goals. In contradistinction to the legislation granting funding for particular programs, there is relatively little legislation concerning regulation of AHCs. Civil rights legislation prohibiting discrimination applies to AHCs. Regulations applied to all hospitals are applied to AHCs as well.

Very little federal legislation precludes AHCs from opting out of relationships with the government. The reason for the close relationship on both sides is that each side has something the other wishes. AHCs have the personnel and facilities to provide the necessary services and meet national policy goals; Congress and the federal agencies have access to resources that AHCs desire.

# References

1. 42 U.S.C.A.

2. 12 U.S.C.A.

3. *Ibid.* Section 1715(z)(7). Mortgage insurance for hospitals. Paragraph (g), subparagraphs (1), (2).

4.  *Ibid.* Section 1715(z)(7). Mortgage insurance for hospitals. Paragraph (a).

5.  Title 42. The Public Health and Welfare. Chapter 6A—Public Health Services. Subchapter V—Health Research and Teaching Facilities and Training of Professional Health Personnel. Part B—Grants and Loan Guarantees and Interest Subsidies for Construction of Teaching Facilities for Medical, Dental, and Other Health Personnel. 42 U.S.C.A. Section 293.

6.  *Ibid.* 42 U.S.C.A. Section 293 (e).

7.  42 U.S.C.A. Section 293(a)(2).

8.  42 U.S.C.A. Section 293(c). Recovery.

9.  42 U.S.C.A. Section 292(b). National Advisory Council on Education for Health Professionals.

10. *Ibid.* 42 U.S.C.A. Section 292(b), paragraph (b). Functions.

11. 42 U.S.C.A. Section 292(b), paragraph (a). Establishment; composition; selection of members. Paragraph (b). Functions.

12. Title 42. The Public Health and Welfare. Chapter 6A—Public Health Service. Subchapter V—Health Research and Teaching Facilities and Training of Professional Health Personnel. Part H—Graduate Medical Education. Section 295(i). Council on Graduate Medical Education 42 U.S.C.A. 295(i).

13. Title 42. The Public Health and Welfare. Chapter 6A—Public Health Service. Subchapter V—Health Research and Teaching Facilities and Training of Professional Health Personnel. Part F—Grants and Contracts for Programs and Projects. Section 295(g). Project Grants for Establishment of Departments of Family Medicine.

14. *Ibid.* 42 U.S.C.A. Section 295(g), paragraph (c). Family Medicine.

15. *Ibid.* 42 U.S.C.A. Section 295(g)(2). Area Health Education.

16. *Ibid.* 42 U.S.C.A. Section 295(g)(1), paragraph (B).

17. *Ibid.* 42 U.S.C.A. Section 295(g)(4).

18. *Ibid.* 42 U.S.C.A. Section 295(g)(9). Geriatric education centers and geriatric training.

19. *Ibid.* 42 U.S.C.A. Section 295(g)(11). Special projects.

20. 42 U.S.C.A., Chapter 6A, Subchapter V, Part G—Programs for Personnel in Health Administration and in Allied Health. Subpart I—Public Health Personnel, Section 295(h). Grants for Graduate Programs in Health Administration.

21. Department of Health and Human Services. Final Funding Categories, Final Review Criteria and Funding Preference for Training Grants for Acquired Immunodeficiency Syndrome (AIDS) Regional Education Training Centers Program (Sept. 8, 1989) 54 FR 37378-01.

22. Rules and Regulations. Department of Health and Human Services. Health Care Financing Administration. 42 CFR, Parts 405,512,413. [BPD-375-F], RIN 0938-AC27. Medicare Program Changes in Payment Policy for Direct Graduate Medical Education costs. 54 FR 40286-01 I. Background.

23. Department of Veteran Affairs. Advisory Commission on the Future Status of Veterans Health Care. Establishment. 55 FR 11503-02.

24. Title 38. Veteran's Benefits. Part VI—Acquisition and Operation of Hospital and Domiciliary Facilities. Procurement and Supply. Leases of Real Property. Subchapter IV—Sharing Medical Facilities, Equipment, and Information. Section 8154. Exchange of Medical Information.

25. Department of Health and Human Services. Centers for Disease Control. [Program Announcement Number 145] National Institute for Occupational Safety and Health; Cooperative Agreement to Enhance the Training of Primary Care Physicians; Availability of Funds for Fiscal Year 1991. 56 FR 41127-01.

26. *Ibid.*

27. Department of Health and Human Services. Program Announcement and Proposed Funding Priorities for Grands for Faculty Development in Family Medicine. 56 FR 29253-01.

*Lois Margaret Nora, MD, JD, is Assistant Dean, Clinical Curriculum, and Assistant Professor, Neurological Sciences, Rush Medical College and Rush-Presbyterian-St. Luke's Medical Center, Chicago, Ill. Brett Eric Reetz, JD, is an attorney with the law firm of Dalton & Dalton, P.C., Burbank, Ill.*

# Chapter 10

# Institutional and Professional Liability in the Academic Health Center

*by Lois Margaret Nora, MD, JD,*
*and Brett Eric Reetz, JD*

**T**he Academic Health Center (AHC) is subject to the same liability concerns as other hospitals. The combination of roles that the AHC has, however, creates liability concerns particular to its type of organization. This chapter will review some of the liability issues that arise as the AHC acts in its roles of health care provider, educator, and researcher.

## The Academic Health Center as Health Care Provider

The AHC provides health care for a number of patient populations. Some patients use the AHC as a primary health care provider because of geographic proximity and/or because of use of the facility by the patient's primary physician. Other patients are referred (or self-refer) to the institution for specialized care that is unavailable in the community hospital setting.

Although no hospital is immune from suits, certain aspects of the AHC may contribute to the likelihood of a liability suit. These include the size of the institution, the make-up of the patient population, the use of students as health care providers, and the relationship between the AHC and its medical staff. Greater numbers of care providers, including students, may increase the potential for miscommunication and error. Referral patients and their families may not have the same sort of long-term relationship with the institution and/or the treating physician that can develop in a primary care setting. The patient population may be sicker, resulting in larger hospital bills and more unfavorable outcomes.

Some of these things are inevitable, given the character of the AHC. Nonetheless, a degree of control over these situations is possible. Risk management strategies geared toward early identification of, and intervention into, potential liability issues will benefit the institution. Although risk management programs are frequently geared toward specific liability concerns, a broader view may be beneficial. Identification of quality issues, even those unlikely to lead to lawsuits, can trigger remedial programs and enhance patient care. Information sharing between risk managers and others involved in continuous quality improvement can be valuable.

Certain aspects of the physician-institution relationship that exists in the AHC deserve comment. Physicians on the staff of the AHC are far more likely to be employees of the institution than are physicians associated with community hospitals. The AHC may be vicariously liable for the negligence of its employee physicians.

Vicarious liability can be established using several legal arguments. *Respondeat superior*, literally translated "let the master answer," is a legal theory that operates under the same principles as principal-agent.[1] The employer-employee ("master-servant") relationship creates an agency relationship between the physician and the AHC when the physician is acting within the scope of his duties. In these instances, physician negligence can be imputed to the AHC employer.

A plaintiff may also proceed on the basis of the legal doctrine of *res ipsa loquitur*, translated to "the thing speaks for itself." In order to use the principle of *res ipsa loquitur*, the plaintiff must show that the injury sustained was of a kind that ordinarily does not occur in the absence of someone's negligence, that it was caused by an agent or instrumentality within the exclusive control of the defendant and/or its servants, and was not due to any voluntary action or contribution on the part of the plaintiff.[2] When the plaintiff can successfully show this, the burden shifts to the defendant to show who or what caused the injury.

Outside the academic setting, a typical result is that various defendants attempt to demonstrate that the others are negligent. The dilemma faced by an AHC in this situation is that all the potential defendants are under its control and frequently are included under the AHC's insurance and indemnification policy. Shifting blame to an employee, physician, or trainee does not avoid AHC responsibility. The AHC can avoid liability in these situations by showing that the injury was caused by something out of its control or by plaintiff's failure to show that a specific breach of the applicable standard of care occurred.

Careful appointment and credentialing systems and ongoing quality assurance review of employee physicians will help minimize liability issues. In the AHC, medical staff appointment and credentialing procedures frequently overlap the faculty appointment process. This generally does not present a problem at the time of initial appointment. The dual review of an applicant may, in fact, result in a more rigorous examination of his or her qualifications.

Problems are more likely to occur at the time of medical staff and/or faculty reappointment. Medical staff reappointments should be done at least every two years and more frequently if the appointment is provisional or probationary.[3] Faculty promotions and reappointments are usually done less frequently. Consequently, medical staff appointment and credentialing should be considered separately from faculty appointment and promotion, even though the two processes may have significant overlap.

Medical staff reappointment and credentialing procedures should emphasize areas of clinical practice pertinent to the practitioner. Faculty appointments and promotions frequently emphasize research, publications, and service to the community and institution. These areas, while certainly important, may have limited relevance to the practitioner's clinical practice.Pressures to meet faculty promotion requirements may contribute to a decrease in the clinical activity of the physician and a gradual loss of skills. Consequently, a strong record for academic promotion does not necessarily translate to an equally strong argument for retention of the clinical privileges initially granted to the practitioner. In a similar vein, faculty tenure should not guarantee continuation of clinical privileges if the practitioner does not remain capable of performing.

Emphasizing the importance of clinical activities will strengthen AHCs in several ways. Practitioners at all levels will be encouraged to remain actively involved in patient care. Faculty promotion committees may reassess the importance of, and the weight given to, patient care activities.

Concern about physician reappointment and credentialing and about quality assurance must extend to nonemployee members of the medical staff. There are two major legal reasons for this. First, hospitals have a duty to use due care in the appointment and credentialing process.[4] If a patient is injured through the negligence of a nonemployee member of the medical staff, the hospital may be liable if it knew or should have known about quality issues involving the physician and did not act accordingly. This liability is independent of any claim that the institution is vicariously liable for the physician's negligence.

A second reason for the hospital to review independent members of the medical staff is because a plaintiff may attempt to establish an agency relationship between the AHC and a physician regardless of whether or not the parties mean for one to exist. In some situations, the question of whether an agency relationship exists between a hospital and a physician is a matter of law. When the question is a matter of law, it can be decided by a judge during pretrial procedures. This only occurs when the evidence presented to the court is subject to only one interpretation. More commonly, the question of the existence and scope of an agency relationship is a question of fact reserved for the jury to decide.

A primary source for determining whether or not an agency relationship exists is written documentation that clearly identifies the intent of the parties. This is not the sole determinant, however. Other facts may lead to a conclusion that an ostensible agency relationship exists between an AHC and a physician, even when the clear intent of both parties is that none exists. Evidence that a jury might consider includes the activities of the physician; his or her duties, responsibilities, and source of income; and the right of the AHC to control the status of the physician.

A jury may work very hard to find an agency relationship between an AHC and a physician when faced with a severely injured plaintiff and an apparently judgment-proof physician. In addition to monitoring individual physician quality, it behooves the AHC to require malpractice insurance at adequate levels for nonemployee members of the medical staff and to ensure that this coverage is maintained.

In addition to having continuous quality improvement and risk management programs throughout the AHC, the institution should be aware of how personnel at affiliated institutions, freestanding clinics, and other facilities represent themselves in relation to the institution. If it is possible that a jury will conclude that an agency relationship exists between the AHC and one of these affiliated bodies, the institution may wish to review quality assurance and risk management practices at these facilities as well.

## The Academic Health Center as Educator

The AHC participates in the education of health professionals with varying levels of expertise in a wide variety of fields. A critical part of the education of health professionals is the apprentice, hands-on training that students get as they assist the health care team in providing care to patients. The AHC is expected to provide an academic environment where students can learn the healing arts while meeting a standard of care at least equivalent to, if not greater than that of, the nonteaching hospital. No special immunities or legal privileges are conferred on the AHC solely because of its role as educator.

Problems that occur related to the AHC's role as educator can be illustrated via a discussion of issues related to medical student and graduate medical student (resident) participation in the delivery of health care in the AHC. Helms and Helms have reviewed litigation involving medical students and residents since 1950.[5-8] Litigation involving medical students, residents and graduate medical education programs have increased over the past generation. The increase in medical student litigation appears to correlate with the increased number of medical students and their increasing debt burden during these years. Medical student litigation predominantly involved issues of medical school admission and dismissal and the financing of medical education. The AHC is less likely to be involved in these cases than the medical college.

Litigation involving residents includes suits about programmatic issues as well as malpractice. Programmatic issues—the organization, support, and administration of residency programs—accounted for slightly more than one-fifth of the resident cases reviewed by Helms and Helms. There has been a sharp increase in the number of these cases brought in the past decade, and academic administration has provided a majority of the cases.

Increases in malpractice litigation involving residents appear to follow national trends and account for the bulk of resident-related litigation. Litigation involving residents revolves around three major issues, frequently in combination--vicarious liability, the standard of care that the resident must meet, and the duty of the institution to supervise the resident. These issues usually arise in the context of a malpractice case, and the AHC is likely to be involved.

One would not expect a medical student or resident to be the sole (or primary) defendant named in a lawsuit. No doubt this correlates to the educational debts and relative poverty of these individuals. A plaintiff gains no compensation, and the plaintiff's attorney gains no contingency fee, by obtaining a judgment against a party who does not have the resources to pay. Therefore, in almost all cases, the ultimate goal of the plaintiff is not to impose liability upon the resident but to reach the institutional "deep pockets" behind him or her.

One way of reaching the AHC's deep pockets is to establish its vicarious liability for the trainee's activities. For the most part, the issues of actual agency and ostensible agency are similar for trainees and employee-physicians. Certain differences do exist, however. Liability issues involving trainees may be complicated by the relationship between the medical college and AHC. The medical college frequently selects and directly employs the resident. The AHC provides the environment in which the resident learns and works. Resident physicians may be agents of a hospital despite being selected and paid by an associated university.[9,10] In fact, two or more entities acting as joint employers or principals may both be held liable for injuries attributable to negligent acts of a single employee or agent.

Disagreement about a resident's relationship to an institution may be particularly acute when one of the institutions involved is a public institution and the other is not. Public institutions, in many cases, have sovereign immunity protection. Sovereign immunity protects the institution from liability for negligent acts. Usually, the immunity remains with the state facility and does not extend to private facilities, even if they are involved in the same training program.[11]

The use of trainees does not, of itself, expose the AHC to liability. A procedure performed properly (including appropriate informed consent) by the most junior member of the health care team subjects the AHC to no liability. A plaintiff will not successfully plead that inadequate care was provided solely because it was administered by a student. In most instances, a specific breach in the standard of care must be proven.

The appropriate standard of care for a resident has been litigated over the years. For many years, the standard identified was that of the "average" resident.[12] What "average" meant was a subject of litigation. For example, a resident was expected to chart information in an appropriate manner but was not expected to overrule the judgment of the supervising physician in an area of medical decision-making.[13] In one case, the court took notice of expert testimony that there is a lack of a uniform standard of care as to resident physicians and that, in fact, there may be variations within one hospital.[13]

Increasingly, there is a tendency to hold care provided by residents to the national standard of care that exists for their specialty. In *McCullough v. Hutzel Hospital*, (276 N.W.2d 569), obstetrician-gynecologists supervised the care of a patient. The specialists did not actually perform tubal ligation surgery on the patient but were responsible for the resident who did. The court found the specialist liable when the patient subsequently became pregnant. The court held that the supervision of the resident constituted the practice of medicine and that care given by a resident should be measured against the supervisor's standard, regardless of who actually provided the hands-on care.

While *McCullough* might be interpreted as encouraging supervision by lesser trained personnel, this would be inappropriate. *McCullough* also does not imply that a resident is or should be as capable in a given procedure as the supervising physician. The case does imply that a supervisor has a duty to make sure that the procedure is done nonnegligently. The basis for holding residents to the national specialty standard of care is based on the expectation that the resident will be supervised and that this supervision will ensure that the patient receives care meeting this standard. This duty of supervision is shared by the AHC, the educational program, and physicians directly involved in the supervision.

Related to this, an injured party may sue an AHC for failure to adequately supervise a trainee. A suit for negligent supervision is different than finding the AHC vicariously liable for the trainee's negligence. It is an independent cause of action against the training institution. The suit asserts that the AHC had a duty to properly supervise the negligent resident, that the AHC failed in its duty to properly supervise the resident, and that this failure proximately caused the injury to the plaintiff.

Suit may be brought when the actions of a single negligent resident result in injury to a patient. Patients may also bring suit against the AHC and other entities for negligence in the supervision of a training program. For example, the governing board of Louisiana State University was successfully sued for negligence in administrating a team approach to health care delivery on a psychiatric ward.[14] Consequently, AHCs and their associated training programs must provide adequate oversight of the training process as well as of the individual care of patients.

## The Academic Health Center as Researcher

In addition to health care provider and educator, the AHC frequently has a significant research mission. This research may be in the basic or clinical sciences. It may involve human subjects who are patients of the institution as well as persons recruited to the institution for research purposes. Unfortunate events demonstrate that abuses in research continue even to the present time.[15,16]

Institutional review boards (IRBs) are mandated by federal law.[17] These Boards are established to ensure that research in conducted in a legal and ethical manner. Specific concerns of the IRB must include adequacy of informed consent that is provided to research subjects, and the risk-benefit ratio of the research to the participants. Other issues to be addressed include equitable selection of subjects and appropriate design of studies. The standards must be particularly rigorous when research will involve incompetent subjects. Meeting standards established by government agencies, including a rigorous IRB, will help avoid legal risks related to research in the institution.

Maintaining confidentiality is another potential problem in the AHC. Research records must avoid revealing a patient's identity. This includes release of personal information specific enough to identify the individual as well as release of the patient's name.

In the AHC, problems with confidentiality are more likely to occur in settings other than formal research studies. Those conducting formal studies are more likely to have a clear awareness of the need for participant privacy after going through IRB approval and other formal steps. It is informal case reports and presentations by faculty to others (both within and outside of the institution) that are more likely to breach confidentiality.

The institution should educate faculty to the importance of maintaining privacy. Patient radiographs and pictures and other elements of presentations should be carefully prepared to delete the patient's name or other identifying characteristics. If this is impossible, the presenter should obtain consent from the patient prior to use of the material.

## Summary

The AHC has multiple roles and many responsibilities. Although fulfillment of these duties may be associated with legal problems, the institution can avoid these problems by meeting appropriate standards of care. Risk management programs to identify potential liability problems and to intervene in these situations, and continuous quality improvement programs designed to continually assess and upgrade institutional activities, can be extremely helpful in avoiding bad outcomes.

## References

1. King, J. *The Law of Medical Malpractice in a Nutshell.* St. Paul, Minn.: West Publishing Co., 1977, pp. 231-2.

2. *Ibid.* pp. 112-3.

3. *Accreditation Manual for Hospitals.* Oak Brook, Ill.: Joint Commission on Accreditation of Healthcare Organizations, 1992, p.58.

4. *Darling v. Charleston Community Memorial Hosp.*, 33 Ill.2d 326, 211 N.E.2d 253, cert denied, 383 U.S. 946 (1966).

5. Helms, L., and Helms, C. "Forty Years of Litigation Involving Medical Students and Their Education. I. General Educational Issues." *Academic Medicine* 66(1):1-7, Jan. 1991.

6. Helms, L., and Helms, C. "Forty Years of Litigation Involving Medical Students and Their Education. II. Issues of Finance." *Academic Medicine* 66(2):71-6, Feb. 1991.

7. Helms, L., and Helms, C. "Forty Years of Litigation Involving Residents and Their Training: I. General Programmatic Issues." *Academic Medicine* 66(11):649-55, Nov. 1991.

8. Helms, L., and Helms, C. "Forty Years of Litigation Involving Residents and Their Training: II. Malpractice Issues. *Academic Medicine* 66(12):718-25, Dec. 1991.

9. *Richter v. Northwestern Memorial Hosp.*, 532 N.E.2d 269 (Ill.App. 1 Dist. 1988).

10. *Shepard v. Sisters of Providence in Oregon,* 89 Or App 579 (1988).

11. *Kelly v. Rossi,* 481 N.E.2d 1340 (Mass. 1985).

12. *Jaar v. University of Miami,* 474 So.2d 239 (Fla.App. 3 Dist. 1988).

13. *Cornell v. State University Hospitals,* 521 N.E.2d 857 (Ohio Ct.Cl. 1987).

14. *Sibley v. Bd. of Sup'rs of Louisiana State U.* 477 So2d 1094 (La. App. 1 Cir 1986).

15. Jones, J. *Bad Blood—The Tuskegee Syphilis Experiment.* New York, N.Y.: The Free Press, 1981.

16. *Hyman v. Jewish Chronic Diseases Hospital,* 206 N.E.2d 338 (1965).

17. Code of Federal Regulations, 45 CFR 46 (1986).

*Lois Margaret Nora, MD, JD, is Assistant Dean, Clinical Curriculum, and Assistant Professor, Neurological Sciences, Rush Medical College and Rush-Presbyterian-St. Luke's Medical Center, Chicago, Ill. Brett Eric Reetz, JD, is an attorney with the law firm of Dalton & Dalton, P.C., Burbank, Ill.*

# Chapter 11

# Cost Management in the Academic Health Center

*by Thomas J. Poulton, MD*

*"A penny saved is two pence clear."*— Benjamin Franklin

*"A billion here, a billion there...after a while that begins to be some real money."*—Everett Dirksen

Limiting the expenditure side of the balance sheet in large organizations is daunting because of the magnitude of aggregate spending. Where does one begin? Fortunately, expenses are dealt with one item at a time and by one person at a time. The more successful efforts to contain costs have occurred in institutions that have made cost containment a top priority. It must be a focus of awareness for every person with the potential to influence the consumption of expendables and the utilization of services, from housekeepers to housestaff and from administrators to admixture aides in the pharmacy.

"Early" attempts at cost containment (circa 1970) were met with considerable resistance, because physicians and health care administrators doubted not only the imperative to reduce medical expenses, but also confronted pragmatic arguments that tended to preserve the status quo.[1,2,3] Specifically, academic medicine in America had traditionally, if not entirely consistently, held that the rights and needs of the individual patient must be placed higher than the collective needs of society.[4,5] That mindset has not been conducive to controlling spending. Today, we realize that cost containment will continue to be forced upon us--brutally perhaps--if we do not embrace it voluntarily.[6-11]

In a milestone article that is now nearly 10 years old, Ginzberg[12] defined medical cost containment as "a reduced inflow of real resources into the health care system without diminution in useful output that would adversely affect the satisfaction of patients or their health status." Viewed at the time by many as doubtfully achievable, experience in the subsequent decade has shown that there was, indeed, a great deal of cost reduction to be accomplished. Platt[13] subsequently articulated six conditions that must be met to achieve cost containment, as defined by Ginzberg:

■ **Higher priced technologies introduced into medicine must produce a clear benefit over existing less costly technologies.**

This mandate conflicts directly with the post-World War II role of the academic health center as *the* site for aggressive development and utilization of technology as it became available from increasingly diverse sectors of the American economy. Integration of increasingly complex imaging techniques and other high-technology diagnostic equipment epitomizes this trend. The role of the academic health center as the developer and champion of such new technologies conflicts directly with the new mandates.[14]

■ **Physicians must exercise self-restraint in utilizing resources.**

This writer remembers vividly during his medicine internship in 1975 that housestaff looked with awe and respect upon the senior residents and attending physicians who created the most extensive lists of orders for diagnostic workups and care of patients. The ability to conceive of unlikely but remotely possible diagnoses and complicated ways to rule them in or out was viewed as the ultimate evidence of the physician's skill and knowledge. New mandates for cost control are incompatible with this tradition. Not only must physicians change behaviors, but, within the academic health center culture, the physician's ability to diagnose incisively, efficiently, and quickly and his or her tolerance for the ambiguity that remains from less than exhaustive diagnostic evaluations must come to be valued, rewarded, and respected as much as the encyclopedic approach was two decades ago. That transition is far from complete.[2]

■ **Outpatient care must be substituted for inpatient care whenever safe and effective.**

Driven aggressively and relentlessly by pressure from third-party payers, we have learned in the past decade that services most never dreamed possible on an outpatient basis are now accomplished routinely. New ways of looking at old problems and solutions must be encouraged to define additional cost-effective approaches in all areas of health care.

■ **Hospitals must reduce ancillary personnel.**

In 1975, it was considered not only appropriate, but also necessary for adequate functioning to have at least 3.5 full-time equivalent personnel for each bed in an academic health center.[15] Budget realities have led to a contemporary ratio of 2.1 to 3.1.[16]

At the same time, changes in utilization of personnel in support of patient care have occurred. Fifteen years ago, it was common in most academic health centers for medical students and junior housestaff to occupy significant portions of their time providing direct patient care and auxiliary services such as transportation, phlebotomy, etc. Changes in expectations and the demands of the medical education marketplace have led to dramatic changes in the frequency with which students and house officers perform such services. Thus, most academic hospitals in the past actually had caregiver-to-patient ratios higher than reported, because, at any given time, there would be as many as several hundred medical students per institution providing the work of scores of full-time equivalent personnel. Today, housestaff and students expect to receive training in institutions where their time will be focused on learning and providing services meaningful in an educational sense, not in service to the hospital.

■ **Duplicate services must be eliminated.**

Perhaps above all else, the public and journalistic eye has focused on duplication of services as symbolic of the inefficiency and waste of past decades. Academic institutions have participated in this duplication extensively. In some areas, academic centers are in direct regional competition with other academic institutions. Everywhere, there is intense town/gown competition that makes it very difficult for the university hospital not to compete by developing service lines and technologies that may exist elsewhere in the region or even within the same community. Strategies must be developed to negotiate effectively with competing institutions those accommodations that enable curtailment of this "technology war."

Unfortunately, such rational and reasoned agreements must be negotiated in an extremely complex social, medical, and legal milieu in which concessions and arrangements that may clearly be in society's and the community's best interests and that will most obviously and directly lead to reductions in regional expenditures for health care technology may ensnare the agreeing institutions in accusations of unfair restraint of trade or of antitrust activities.

■ **Widespread patient education should be undertaken to encourage healthy life-styles.**

Self-inflicted disease and disability remain overwhelming problems in America. Earlier concerns about the economic and health costs of inactivity, smoking, and drug abuse will be dwarfed in the coming decade by the social, medical, and societal costs of HIV-associated illness. Any effective educational efforts must be developed within a society that has long valued individual rights and prerogatives highly. Mass education funded by the government is viewed suspiciously in America as potential indoctrination and as a dangerous precedent.

The importance of the rights of the individual has been translated traditionally in a very practical sense within academic health centers as providing the very best medical care possible for each and every patient, regardless of the cost involved. The collective needs of society have been viewed as secondary and as an external constraint not operating on the individual patient-physician relationship. Clearly, that is changing, and it is so fundamental a change that it may well be the emerging operational distillation of the paradigm-shift in American health care. Whether that change is desirable is being debated.[17]

Although a broad discussion of the imperative for cost reduction is beyond the scope of this chapter, it is clear that the technological and other successes of contemporary American health care institutions have come at a great price. More than 12 percent of the gross national product presently goes to health care[18] and that proportion will increase to 16 percent by the year 2000.[19] The mandate for change comes not only from the federal government, but now increasingly from state governments through Medicaid programs as well as from private insurers. The question is not "when?" but only "how?" substantial reductions in the proportion of national spending on health care will be accomplished.

Some cost containment occurs involuntarily in academia; when revenues are not available, expenditures *must* be cut. Particularly susceptible are the direct and indirect expenses for medical education, especially the expenses of advanced fellowship training. Strategies to protect and increase revenues are not reviewed in this chapter, but they are of great importance. Broad strategies to promote cooperation with health care insurers and purchasers (industry) are also crucial.

Cooperative cost management ventures, although certainly rational intuitively, also involve threats to the basic structure of the university. "Cooperation" often carries with it the price of compromise of autonomy, one of the cornerstones of the university for centuries. Involvement of for-profit corporations in the operations of academic health centers and the expansion of private corporate funding for research demand careful consideration and monitoring of their impact on the role of the academic health center.

Vanselow has reviewed the financial status of U.S. teaching hospitals.[8] Total margins for major academic centers have declined sharply in the past decade. This is generally attributed to the present combination of prospective payment and the high level of uncompensated and undercompensated care that most academic centers are obliged to provide.

Thus, while the "big" issues of federal funding for health care, the differential distribution of that funding to academic and private institutions, the participation by private insurers in the indirect expenses of medical education, and other equally important issues are crucially important,[20,21] the remainder of this chapter focuses on "micro" strategies to deal with cost control. Many of the cost-reducing strategies employed in academic health centers have been used in the past decade by other American businesses facing similar economic pressures. Simply put, the successful academic health center must be run as any other business, with top-to-bottom education in fundamental management principles and a virtually evangelistic approach to economizing in ways that improve efficiency without compromising the overall mission of the institution.

An analysis produced in 1989 by the Health-Care Advisory Board in Washington, D.C., identified cost-management strategies applicable to academic as well as private hospitals.[22] These strategies include the restructuring of departments and work routines in creative ways to eliminate excess personnel. Although all managers are aware of "economies of scale," the implications of the reality have not previously been applied creatively and aggressively to academic health centers.

Acknowledgement of the benefits of such economies of scale includes creative combinations of small departments into larger units. Such restructuring affords opportunities for cross-training, elimination of management positions, and reductions of excess FTEs. The combination of multiple specialty-based intensive care units into large integrated critical care units is an example directly relevant to the academic setting. In the past, neurosurgeons, cardiac surgeons, cardiologists, and others have made a case for their need for units dedicated strictly to their own specialty's patients. Although arguably meaningful in an educational sense, the creation of many such (usually small) units within a large academic institution inevitably leads to increasing and unnecessary numbers of supervisory personnel and expenses associated with fluctuating census within individual units. Merging such units into "mega-ICUs" provides greater predictability in total census, which provides the opportunity to minimize the total staff commitment required. Further, the elimination of head nurse positions for each small ICU enables the realization of substantial savings in management costs.

The same report concluded that most hospitals in the mid- to late 1980s suffered from top-heavy management structures. In this regard, the academic institution must follow the private sector to remain competitive. A consensus view is that hospitals should have no more than four management levels—president or CEO, vice-president, department director, and supervisor or head nurse. Delegation must be more complete and more effective, and the front-line patient caregivers must be trusted to appropriately apply their skills to implement institutional policies and procedures.

There is growing disillusionment with and skepticism about the effectiveness of medical cost-containment efforts in general.[23-25] The consensus view seems to hold that continued unrestrained public demand, coupled with the continuing largely unrestrained development of increasingly sophisticated and expensive technology, will continue to drive costs up until some "major event" occurs. We must now believe that the major event will be some form of systematic rationing of specific types of care. Regardless of what ultimately precipitates the "major event" to change the manner in which resources are allocated, it is clear that academic institutions that strive to minimize expenses while maximizing the quality of care provided will be positioned best for whatever changes that appear.

Reductions in the number of inpatient days per admission (length of stay, LOS) were one of the key targets of federal prospective payment strategies. Although a 1986 study found that approximately one fourth of hospital admissions and one third of hospital days may have been unnecessary,[26] evidence exists that reductions that *can* be made *have* been made.[27] Modest additional decrements in LOS may be realized using a recently developed tool to assist the teaching hospital in identifying the sources of unnecessary hospital days.[28]

Needless to say, virtually any cost-containing effort used in any hospital can be adapted for use in a teaching setting. Such efforts include not only those detailed above, but such strategies as taking advantage of purchases of reconditioned rather than new equipment,[29] using bar coding within the hospital to facilitate the assignment of charges and the control of inventories,[30] using less expensive off-site storage for medical center documents,[31] carefully reviewing the effect of any new technology on the bottom line,[32] and reevaluating reusable rather than disposable supplies.[33,34]

Specific studies of strategies to reduce costs in academic settings can generally be grouped into those that have attempted to change physician test-ordering behaviors, those that have attempted to change physician prescribing behaviors (especially of antibiotics), and those that have looked more globally at all or many costs associated with certain product lines (such as a specific surgical program).

Attempts to change the ordering of drugs for inpatients by physicians in university medical centers have included a variety of strategies.[35-37] What has come to be known as "academic detailing"[38] has been successful in a small number of medical centers for a very limited number of drugs, but the process is extremely labor-intensive, tending to offset the savings realized.

Antibiotic formulary restrictions have been adopted frequently to attempt to control expenditures for antibiotics. Interestingly, one study found such a restriction of cefotaxime was actually associated with an *increase* in usage of that drug.[39] Other institutions have been able to restrict expenditures by combining restrictions in the formulary with inhospital education of physicians.[40,41] Nickman et al.[42] effectively reduced the duration of prophylactic postoperative antibiotic administration through institutional enforcement of automatic stop orders in accordance with recommendations from the literature. Durbin produced similar results by combining formulary restrictions with a prescription system that required physicians to state whether each specific antibiotic prescription was for prophylactic, empiric, or therapeutic use.[43]

Barnes Hospital, affiliated with the Washington University School of Medicine, studied the effects of formulary restrictions on expenditures as well as crude indices of outcome (length of stay and mortality).[44] The program resulted in annual savings in excess of $300,000, with no discernible impact on morbidity and mortality. Moreover, an analysis after the onset of controls revealed that antibiotics were prescribed more appropriately after the formulary restrictions than before. Significantly, this program depended fundamentally not only on formulary restriction but also on a tactfully conducted educational process of direct consultation by infectious disease experts whenever requests for permission to use restricted antibiotics occurred. This was embraced readily if not enthusiastically because of the implicit educational value for housestaff and attending physicians.

McCloskey et al.[45] found in 1984 that approximately 55 percent of teaching hospitals already had formulary restrictions on cephalosporin usage. Obviously, many academic institutions believe it appropriate to restrict usage of certain antibiotics. Whether most such restrictions are placed with the intent of improving clinical practice or of containing costs, however, is not clear.

One year earlier, Klapp and Ramphal[46] found similar restrictions on broader categories of antibiotics in place at 57 percent of 108 university hospitals. In that study, cost was most often given as the stimulus for instituting the restrictions. Interestingly, no evidence was presented suggesting that the restriction was, in fact, effective in cutting expense.

DeTorres and White[41] demonstrated a cost saving of approximately $15,000 per year from the imposition of formulary restrictions for aminoglycosides in a teaching hospital. The impact on quality of care was not evaluated in this study, and long-term follow-up to confirm any lasting benefits was not done. Somewhat similar studies by Nickman et al.[42] and by Abramowitz et al.[47] suffered from similar limitations.

Laboratory services may represent as much as a quarter of total hospital costs and have been increasing at the rate of approximately 15 percent per year.[48,49] Further, in the academic setting, as much as half of laboratory services may be unnecessary or suboptimal.[50-53] Widely varying strategies of incentives, penalties, educational initiatives, and programs of administrative oversight of laboratory service ordering have produced results that have often been poor and, when positive, difficult to maintain over time.[54-59] Most such studies have had the benefits of documented cost savings compromised to some extent by the labor-intensive nature of physician involvement necessary to achieve ongoing benefit. Spiegel and Shapiro developed a program at UCLA that was designed specifically to minimize the need for expensive ongoing physician administrative time to maintain the program.[54] In that study, orders for inappropriate initial or admission chest x-rays decreased by 22 percent, and inappropriate orders for "routine" urinalysis, chest x-rays, and differential leukocyte counts decreased by 23 percent, 30 percent, and 46 percent, respectively.

Gross and Van Antwerpen at the University of Medicine and Dentistry of New Jersey in Newark showed a substantial decrease in inappropriate ordering of blood cultures during a period of study.[55] Although the projected annual cost savings was substantial, the net benefit was illusory, for follow-up revealed that without intensive and continuous input, inappropriate ordering (and increased expense) recurred shortly after the period of study. Neu addressed the same issue editorially but offered no solution other than increased efforts to educate physicians.[60]

Can educational efforts really work to alter physicians' test-ordering behaviors? Schroeder et al.[52] believe not. They found that both a lecture series and a system of chart audits with feedback to the physicians involved in excessive use of any of nine laboratory tests and nursing interventions brought little benefit. In this investigation, most effort was focused on first-year house officers. It is possible that entry-level resident physicians have less impact on what is ordered than believed. Perhaps the same approach, focused more on senior residents and attending physicians, would have a more desirable effect.

Other well-conceived studies have generally found that interventions to change test ordering behaviors are expensive and that their positive effects are generally short-lived. Sommers et al. investigated the impact that doctors and nurses could have in reducing expenses associated with a specific service line (in this case, total hip arthroplasty).[61] Three orthopedic surgeons and three nurses met 20 times during a two-year period and functioned primarily as a "brainstorming" group to consider ideas that might effect cost savings. The task force identified several areas where costs could be limited: eliminating excessive preoperative laboratory testing, eliminating wasted time in the operating room, and decreasing unnecessarily lengthy postoperative stays. During the study period, average hospital expenses decreased by over $2,000 per procedure, almost a 10 percent reduction.

Cohen and Jones in 1982 assessed the availability of cost information as a means of influencing physician test ordering.[62] They found that test utilization fell during the period of study but remained lower after the experimental period only on those teams having a leader committed to the effectiveness of the program.

One can review the results of the studies above and mistakenly believe either that interventions are hopeless or that they are relatively simple. In truth, the ease with which change in human behavior occurs depends on many institution-specific factors. If one views changes in behaviors effecting costs in the broader context of change in general, it is well established that the least disruptive and longest-lasting changes occur in organizations with strong and consistent leadership for change present at the highest levels and throughout the management structure.

In that regard, many of the discouraging results of early attempts to influence clinical behaviors to minimize expenditure require reevaluation. The environment for change in cost management in the academic health center is not the same as it was even five years ago. It is categorically different from that which existed a decade ago, when more research on cost containment was being published than has been the case recently. A new generation of residents has recently completed undergraduate medical education during which cost has been discussed, for the first time, as an integral part of many portions of the curriculum. Further, many faculty members who 10 years ago vigorously resisted economically motivated changes in clinical behavior have come to see change not only as necessary, but also as desirable. Thus, contemporary attempts to change behaviors will occur in a very different setting from those earlier studies cited above. Indeed, in many academic centers, a significant percentage of educational conferences include relevant financial data to assist attendings, housestaff, and medical students to understand the financial implications of their clinical decisions. Such routine discussions, one must imagine, will provide a more favorable substrate for further interventions for change. A few recent studies are exemplary in demonstrating that high-quality research can answer questions about cost *and* quality simultaneously.[63,64]

Ironically, the very financial constraints that mandate tight cost management also limit the funds available to conduct research on the impact of attempts to create effective changes. Urgently needed is funding for studies *today* of what is and is not effective *today* in cost management in the academic center. All levels of government, as well as commercial insurers, have a legitimate interest in such studies and should assist in funding them.

Ultimately, academic managers must believe that they will be rewarded for providing efficient, cost-managed, high-quality care. The present health care system in this country does not necessarily provide that reward.[65] Cost management in the academic health center must mature hand-in-hand with the evolution of a national system of health care financing that recognizes and rewards efficiency coupled with excellence. When that ability to recognize excellence develops, we *must* be delivering it.

## References

1.  Myers, L., and Schroeder, S. "Physician Use of Services for the Hospitalized Patient: A Review, with Implications for Cost Containment." *Milbank Memorial Fund Quarterly* 59(4):481-507, Fall 1981.

2.  Eisenberg, J., and Williams, S. "Cost Containment and Changing Physicians' Practice Behavior: Can the Fox Learn to Guard the Chicken Coop?" *JAMA* 246(19):2195-201, Nov. 13, 1981.

3.  McPhee, S., and others. "The Costs and Risks of Medical Care: An Annotated Bibliography for Clinicians and Educators." *Western Journal of Medicine* 137(2):145-61, Aug. 1982.

4.  Harrison, D. "Cost Containment Issues in Medicine: Why Cardiology?." *American Journal of Cardiology* 56(5):10C-15C, Aug. 23, 1985.

5.  Reinhardt, U. "Future Trends in the Economics of Medical Practice and Care. *American Journal of Cardiology* 56(5):50C-59C, Aug. 23, 1985.

6.  Knoebel, S. "Cardiology by the Numbers and Cost-Containment." *American Journal of Cardiology* 61(13):1112-5, May 1, 1988.

7.  Reagan, M. "Health Care Rationing: What Does It Mean?" *New England Journal of Medicine* 319(17):1149-51, Oct. 27, 1988.

8.  Vanselow, N. "The Financial Status of U.S. Teaching Hospitals." *Academic Medicine* 65(9):560-1, Sept. 1990.

9.  Knoebel, S., and Dittus, R. "ACC Anniversary Seminar. Introduction." *Journal of the American College of Cardiology* 13(1):1-2, Jan. 1989.

10. Ginzberg, E. "A Hard Look at Cost Containment." *New England Journal of Medicine* 316(18):1151-4, April 30, 1987.

11. Relman, A. "Is Rationing Inevitable?" *New England Journal of Medicine* 322(25):1809-10, June 21, 1990.

12. Ginzberg, E. "Sounding Board. Cost Containment—Imaginary and Real." *New England Journal of Medicine* 308(20):1220-4, May 19, 1983.

13. Platt, R. "Sounding Board: Cost Containment--Another View." *New England Journal of Medicine* 309(12):726-30, Sept. 22, 1983.

14. Ross, R., and Johns, M. "Changing Environment and the Academic Medical Center: The Johns Hopkins School of Medicine." *Academic Medicine* 64(1):1-6, Jan. 1989.

15. American Hospital Association. *Hospital Statistics*. Chicago, Ill.: AHA, 1975.

16. Sear, A. "Comparison of Efficiency and Profitability of Investor-Owned Multihospital Systems with Not-for-Profit Hospitals." *Health Care Management Review* 16(3):31-7, Spring 1991.

17. Sulmasy, D. "Physicians, Cost Control, and Ethics." *Annals of Internal Medicine* 116(11):920-6, June 1, 1992.

18. Office of National Cost Estimates. "National Health Expenditures, 1988." *Health Care Financing Review* 11(4):1-41, Summer 1990.

19. Rich, S. Health Costs to Consume 16% of GNP by 2000, Agency Says." *Washington Post* Aug. 24, 1991, p. A2.

20. Page, L. "Teaching Hospitals Forced to Redesign Themselves." *American Medical News* 35(22):3,57, June 8, 1992.

21. MacKenzie, T., and others. "Indirect Costs of Teaching in Canadian Hospitals." *Canadian Medical Association Journal* 144(2):149-52, Jan. 15, 1991.

22. Burda, D. "Report Card Grades Cost-Saving Strategies." *Modern Healthcare* 19(52):50, Dec. 29, 1989.

23. Eddy, D. "Clinical Decision Making: From Theory to Practice. Connecting Value and Costs. Whom Do We Ask. and What Do We Ask Them?" *JAMA* 264(13):1737-9, Oct. 3, 1990.

24. Eddy, D. "What Care Is Essential'? What Services Are 'Basic'?" *JAMA* 265(6):782-8, Feb. 13, 1991.

25. Callahan, D. *What Kind of Life: The Limits of Medical Progress*. New York, N.Y.:Simon & Schuster, Inc., 1990, p. 191.

26. Siu, A., and others. "Inappropriate Use of Hospitals in a Randomized Trial of Health Insurance Plans." *New England Journal of Medicine* 315(20):1259-66, Nov. 13, 1986.

27. Schwartz, W., and Mendelson, D. "Hospital Cost Containment in the 1980s. Hard Lessons Learned and Prospects for 1990s" *New England Journal of Medicine* 324(15):1037-42, April 11, 1991.

28. Selker, H., and others. "The Epidemiology of Delays in a Teaching Hospital. The Development and Use of a Tool that Detects Unnecessary Hospital Days." *Medical Care* 27(2):112-29, Feb. 1989.

29. Sitcer, G. "Surgical Table Rebuilding a Cost Containment Option." *Journal of Healthcare Materiel Management* 8(4):40-4, May-June 1990.

30. Holmes, L. "A Survey of Bar Coding in Canadian Teaching Hospitals." *Dimensions in Health Services* 64(7):23-5, Oct. 1987.

31. Sommers, R., and others. "Off-Site Storage--Move It!" *Journal of Healthcare Material Management* 8(1):26,28-30, 32 passim, Jan. 1990.

32. Maier, R. "'New Math' Teaches Lessons of Reducing Costs of Care." *Modern Healthcare* 19(43):58, Oct. 27, 1989.

33. Moran, E. "Hospitals Look for Savings in Unusual Places." *Hospitals* 63(24):53, Dec. 20, 1989.

34. Summers, J. "Overindulgence and Cost Containment." *Journal of Healthcare Materiel Management* 8(5):68-70, July 1990.

35. Frazier, L., and others. "Can Physician Education Lower the Cost of Prescription Drugs? A Prospective Controlled Trial." *Annals of Internal Medicine* 115(2):116-21, July 15, 1991.

36. Klein, L., and others. "Effect of Physician Tutorials on Prescribing Patterns of Graduate Physicians." *Journal of Medical Education* 56(6):504-11, June 1981.

37. Clapham, C., and others. "Economic Consequences of Two Drug-Use Control Systems in a Teaching Hospital." *American Journal of Hospital Pharmacy* 45(11):2329-40, Nov. 1988.

38. Avorn, J., and Soumerai, S. "Improving Drug-Therapy Decisions through Education Outreach. A Randomized Controlled Trial of Academically Based 'Detailing.'" *New England Journal of Medicine* 308(24):1457-63, June 16, 1983.

39. DeVito, J., and John, J. "Effect of Formulary Restriction of Cefotaxime Usage." *Archives of Internal Medicine* 145(6):1053-6, June 1985.

40. Recco, R., and others. "Antibiotic Control in a Municipal Hospital." *JAMA* 241(21):2283-6, May 25, 1979.

41. DeTorres, O., and White, R. "Effect of Aminoglycoside-Use Restrictions on Drug Cost." *American Journal of Hospital Pharmacy* 41(6):1137-9, June 1984.

42. Nickman, N., and others. "Medical Committee Enforcement of Policy Limiting Postsurgical Antibiotic Use." *American Journal of Hospital Pharmacy* 41(10):2053-6, Oct. 1984.

43. Durbin, W., and others. "Improved Antibiotic Usage Following Introduction of a Novel Prescription System." *JAMA* 246(16):1796-800, Oct. 16, 1981.

44. Woodward, R., and others. "Antibiotic Cost Savings from Formulary Restrictions and Physician Monitoring in a Medical-School-Affiliated Hospital." *American Journal of Medicine* 83(5):817-23, Nov. 1987.

45. McCloskey, W., and others. "Cephalosporin-Use Restrictions in Teaching Hospitals." American Journal of Hospital Pharmacy 41(11):2359-62, Nov. 1984.

46. Klapp, D., and Ramphal, R. "Antibiotic Restriction in Hospitals Associated with Medical Schools." *American Journal of Hospital Pharmacy* 40(11):1957-60, Nov. 1983.

47. Abramowitz, P., and others. "Use of Clinical Pharmacists to Reduce Cefamandole, Cefoxitin, and Ticarcillin Costs." *American Journal of Hospital Pharmacy* 39(7):1176-80, July 1982.

48. Fineberg, H. "Clinical Chemistries: The High Cost of Low-Cost Diagnostic Test." In Altman, S., and Blendon, R., Eds. *Medical Technologies: The Culprit behind Health Care Costs?* Washington, D.C.: U.S. Government Printing Office, 1979, pp. 144-65. (DHEW publication no. [PHS]79-3216).

49. Conn, R. "Clinical Laboratories: Profit Center, Production Industry or Patient-Care Resource?" *New England Journal of Medicine* 298(8):422-7, Feb. 23, 1978.

50. Eisenberg, J., and Williams, S. "Limited Usefulness of the Proportion of Tests with Normal Results in Review of Diagnostic Services Utilization." *Clinical Chemistry* 29(12):2111-3, Dec. 1983.

51. Williams, S., and Eisenberg, J. "A Controlled Trial to Decrease the Unnecessary Use of Diagnostic Tests." *Journal of General Internal Medicine* 1(1):8-13, Jan.-Feb. 1986.

52. Schroeder, S., and others. "Use of Laboratory Tests and Pharmaceuticals. Variation among Physicians and Effect of Cost Audit on Subsequent Use." *JAMA* 225(8):969-73, Aug. 20, 1973.

53. Dixon, R., and Laszlo, J. "Utilization of Clinical Chemistry Services by Medical House Staff. An Analysis." *Archives of Internal Medicine* 134(6):1064-7, Dec. 1974.

54. Spiegel, J., and others. "Changing Physician Test Ordering in a University Hospital." *Archives of Internal Medicine* 149(3):549-53, March 1989.

55. Gross, P., and others. "Use and Abuse of Blood Cultures: Program to Limit Use." *American Journal of Infection Control* 16(3):114-7, June 1988.

56. Grossman, R. "A Review of Physician Cost-Containment Strategies for Laboratory Testing." *Medical Care* 21(8):783-802, Aug. 1983.

57. Martin, A., and others. "A Trial of Two Strategies to Modify the Test-Ordering Behavior of Medical Residents." *New England Journal of Medicine* 303(23):1330-6, Dec. 4, 1980.

58. Marton, K., and others. "Modifying Test-Ordering Behavior in the Outpatient Medical Clinic. A Controlled Trial of Two Educational Interventions." *Archives of Internal Medicine* 145(5):816-21, May 1985.

59. Eisenberg, J. "An Educational Program to Modify Laboratory Use by House Staff." *Journal of Medical Education* 52(7):578-81, July 1977.

60. Neu, H. "Cost Effective Blood Cultures--Is It Possible or Impossible to Modify Behavior?" *Infection Control* 7(1):32-3, Jan. 1986.

61. Sommers, L., and others. "Clinician-Directed Hospital Cost Management for Total Hip Arthroplasty Patients." *Clinical Orthopedics* (258):168-75, Sept. 1990.

62. Cohen, D., and others. "Does Cost Information Availability Reduce Physician Test Usage? A Randomized Clinical Trial with Unexpected Findings." *Medical Care* 20(3):286-92, March 1982.

63. Steinberg, E., and others. "Safety and Cost Effectiveness of High-Osmolality as Compared with Low-Osmolality Contrast Material in Patients Undergoing Cardiac Angiography." *New England Journal of Medicine* 326(7):425-30, Feb. 13, 1992.

64. Barrett, B., and others. "A Comparison of Nonionic, Low-Osmolality Radiocontrast Agents with Ionic, High-Osmolality Agents during Cardiac Catheterization." *New England Journal of Medicine* 326(7):431-6, Feb. 13, 1992.

65. McClure, W. "Buying Right: Will Good Medicine Drive out Bad?" *Psychiatric Hospital* 19(2):57-62, Spring 1988.

*Thomas J. Poulton, MD, is Chair, Department of Anesthesiology, St. Francis Hospital and Medical Center, Topeka, Kansas, and Adjunct Professor of Anesthesiology, Creighton University School of Medicine, Omaha, Nebraska.*

# Chapter 12

# Information Systems in Academic Health Centers

*by Paul R. Vegoda and William F. Bria, MD*

T he academic health center is an extremely complex structure from the point of view of information collection and exchange. The three major missions of the academic health center—the provision of patient care, medical research, and medical education—while complementary in nature, generate a profusion of interdepartmental and intrainstitutional information issues that essentially revolve around the ownership of data. Because information is generated by hospital departments, hospital-based clinical departments, clinical departments, private practice plans, the schools, and research laboratories and because significant information exchange is required, integration of information becomes both a technological and a diplomatic tour de force (figure 1, page 144).

The information systems of the academic health center, and there are myriad centralized and departmental systems that must be able to communicate with each other, must support all three missions. These systems must contain corporate and departmental administrative and financial management information, including:

- Admissions, discharge, and transfer, usually referred to as ADT but sometimes called patient management.

- Patient billing and patient accounting (both corporate hospital billing and departmental physician billing).

- General ledger and cost accounting.

- Personnel management.

- Inventory management and operations support systems.

- Ancillary departmental systems, such as laboratory and radiology information systems.

- Clinical systems that support physician order entry and results reporting and longitudinal medical records.

- Clinic appointment scheduling systems that provide for resource and patient scheduling.

- Medical record tracking systems to ensure that the location of each medical record is tracked and known.

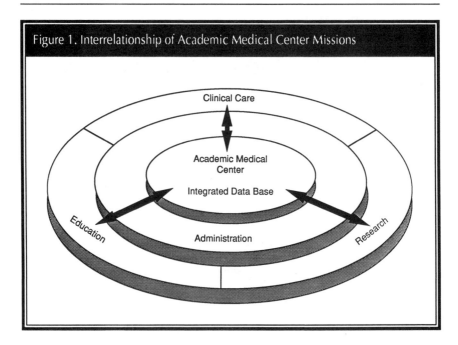

Figure 1. Interrelationship of Academic Medical Center Missions

- Nursing support systems, such as care planning, acuity measurement, recording and charting of vital signs, and automatic generation of medical administration reports.

- Physician support systems that generate patient reports for rounds and that allow on-line generation of progress reports and discharge summaries.

For a system of this complexity to be successful, there must be a strategic blueprint for success:

- Open networking standards that will allow interoperability among different vendor platforms must be implemented. Without an underlying network that facilitates communications among the various departmental and corporate components, the academic health center information system cannot succeed as an integrated system.

- There must be an integrated database that serves as the repository for information that is developed by corporate, ancillary, and departmental systems. The integrated database allows the academic health center information system to be patient-centered, as opposed to being solely department-oriented.

- The system must be patient-centered. That means that a physician can sign onto the system and automatically have displayed a list of his or her patients. When a patient is selected, all pertinent information is available, i.e., order status and results from all ancillaries. As systems become more sophisticated, progress notes and discharge summaries will also be available. A patient-centered system also allows for development of a longitudinal medical record that follows the patient's progress as both inpatient and outpatient.

■ The system must be user-centered—easy to use and mirroring the thought processes of the user. For instance, it should have customized physician order sets so that when the physician signs on to the system, his or her specific ordering requirements are generated on the workstation. Automatically generated nursing care plans should also be an integrated part of the system.

■ The system must be a distributed system. This means that while the corporate system maintains the integrated database, departmental systems continue to meet the needs of the individual departments. Departmental systems are operated by the departments, with orders and results flowing through the integrated database.

■ Ideally, the clinical data gathered from the patient care information system will be extracted into a research database that will support the research and education missions of the medical center.

These six strategic goals form the basis for the development of a medical center information system that ensures that the varied information needs of a very diverse population can be met. In today's medical center world, there are generally three levels of information systems.

The corporate or centralized system, usually managed by the university hospital, maintains corporate systems, such as payroll, personnel, patient billing, general ledger, inventory management, medical records, and frequently a patient care information system. The corporate system is usually mainframe-based. It requires a computer facility and is used as the repository and central distribution point for corporate information.

The hospital information services department maintains the applications on the mainframe computer, develops and implements new applications, and is charged with responsibility for maintaining the networks throughout the medical center. Because the networks act like the information veins and arteries of the medical center's information system, maintaining this vital link is a very high priority. Whatever networking scheme is implemented, it is essential that all the network elements meet similar standards so that they are compatible. (An example of compatible networks would be the implementation of TCP/IP on a fiberoptic FDDI backbone. This approach will allow users of differing technologies to interconnect, i.e., Apple Macintosh workstations on an Appletalk local area network (LAN) can communicate with IBM PS/2 workstations on Banyan or Novell LANs. Departments on a DEC VAX system using Ethernet will be able to communicate with other vendors' equipment on a Token Ring LAN.)

Departmental systems, the second level, are usually based on a minicomputer and are associated with a local area network throughout the department. Departmental systems are used for such applications as budgeting, physician billing (or input to a centralized physician billing system), residency tracking, departmental electronic mail (e-mail), and word processing. There are many highly specialized departmental systems, such as laboratory information systems; radiology information systems; radiation oncology treatment planning; operating room scheduling; and various image storage and tracking systems, such as in nuclear medicine; physiological monitoring for the intensive care units, operating rooms, and emergency department; and medical record imaging.                   .

In addition to the work described above, departmental LANs are frequently used in support of individual researchers. The advantage is that the researcher can take advantage of the availability of his or her own intelligent workstation as required, use departmental word processing and e-mail facilities in support of that research and other departmental activities, and then take advantage of the mainframe network connections for intensive computing requirements.

The third level is desktop computing using an intelligent workstation. There are three basic categories of intelligent workstations, each with its own adherents—Apple Macintosh, IBM PS/2 and clones, and UNIX-driven. Because an integrated system requires that all components be able to communicate, this mixture of incompatible hardware and software complicates communication. Because each workstation type serves a different need, the use of each is absolutely justified. Strict adherence to a networking standard is essential to ensure that everyone will be able to communicate.

## Supporting the Three Missions

### Patient Care

A university system engenders creative thinking and solutions. The diversity of solutions to problems extends to computers and information systems. Certainly, without this diversity, there would be little progress in the discovery of new and better ways to use computers.

It is precisely because of this diversity that academic health centers may have difficulty with integrated information systems. Successful integrated patient care information systems demand establishment of operation and communication standards that are problematic in the academic setting. However, the current external pressures of regulatory agencies and financial constraints have changed the environment even in university medical centers. In addition, federal grant funds have diminished over the past several years, making clinical operations even more important to the financial health and support of academic health centers. Therefore, the current strategic position in academic health centers is to reexamine the efficiency and effectiveness of patient care operations. This review has included total quality strategies directed at improving the quality of health care services and at more consistent performance relative to quality standards. Therefore, many academic health centers have or are now in the process of considering how technology, in the form of patient care information systems (PCIS), can help them meet their own quality goals.

A PCIS is the core clinical computing application in the strategic plan of academic health center information systems (figure 2, page 147). The PCIS is an integrated communication system handling all patient order entry and results reporting duties for every area of the medical center. As the common communication link between all departments, it acts as the electronic chart for dialogue between health care providers, educators, and researchers. The improved organization and legibility of the electronic charge enhances these communications significantly, which, in turn, improves the consistency and the quality of the care delivered. As indicated in figure 2, the PCIS is tightly integrated into departmental information systems, bringing together all necessary information for the process of patient care. Additionally, because the PCIS is used directly by clinicians, quality assurance information is closely integrated into the ordering portion of the PCIS to assist the clinician in making the best medical decision prospectively.

To be successful, the PCIS must operate according to the logic of clinical practice. The PCIS should support, enhance, and improve the clinician's ability to carry on daily duties in the climate of increasing regulatory and financial demands. Figure 3, below, shows a common clinical decision process carried out by physicians literally dozens of times every day. A patient's result is checked, and, based on this information, a new hypothesis/problem is considered, requiring further

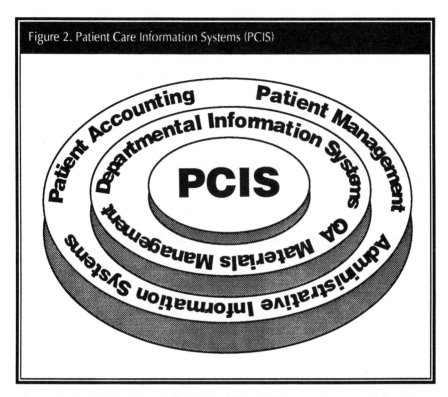

Figure 2. Patient Care Information Systems (PCIS)

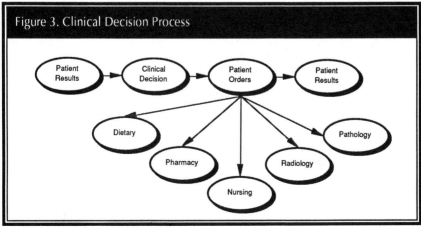

Figure 3. Clinical Decision Process

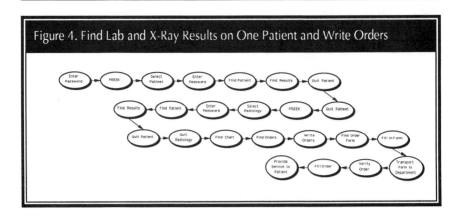

Figure 4. Find Lab and X-Ray Results on One Patient and Write Orders

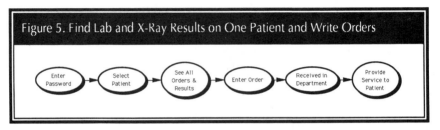

Figure 5. Find Lab and X-Ray Results on One Patient and Write Orders

orders. These orders include a constellation of all the available services in the medical center. The orders are clustered according to the problem being considered rather than along strict departmental lines. From these investigations, further data are obtained and converted into information by the responsible physician. Figure 4, above, shows the process of reviewing results from radiology and laboratory departments using a nonintegrated computer system. The number of steps and the division of information are illogical in terms of the core process of patient care. This sort of PCIS would not effectively or efficiently serve the clinician.

Figure 5, above, shows the same process using an integrated PCIS. Here, the clinician sees a listing of his or her patients automatically, selects a patient, and then immediately retrieves all relevant information at the same time. The data are patient-centered in this model. Additionally, the ordering process is integrated into the same process as results retrieval, eliminating transport of paper requisitions and subsequently allowing the department to communicate directly and interactively with the ordering clinician regarding the requirements for tests and procedures. Because electronic communication between the ordering clinician and the service department is instantaneous, patient care is provided rapidly and efficiently.

The major functional components of a PCIS are:

■ Physician order entry.

■ Integrated results reporting.

■ Communications.

■ Patient scheduling.

- Physician reminders.

- Long-term patient record.

- Concurrent medical education.

- The primary feeding system for a research information system.

Physician order entry embodies two important components: direct physician use and integrated ordering logic. Direct physician use implies that the PCIS is found sufficiently useful and usable if it is integrated into daily patient care rounds by the physician. This capability requires rapid system operation (usually subsecond response time) and intelligence of system operation that make the required change in practice worth the effort. Workflow studies dating back to the early 1970s[1] have shown that physicians will become impatient and will discontinue using computers when information is present less than or equal to 1 second per screen change. Although there are as many styles of clinical rounding as there are physicians doing it, there are several important logical constructs that a PCIS must emulate to be successful:

- **Last in First out Logic**—The most common information pursued is the results from the last written orders.

- **Random Access to Orders from Results**—Ordering does not occur according to department boundaries or other uniform structures. It occurs in response to the clinician's identification of patient problems and to the need for the physician to act. The stimuli for this need to act come from patient examination, conversation with consultants, and test results. Because the PCIS is the main resulting information instrument, it must allow the clinician to order while reviewing previous results and then to continue results review where he or she last left off.

- **Facilitation of Good Clinical Decision Making, Not Control of Physician Behavior**—When a PCIS is first introduced, there is a strong temptation on the part of clinical departments to use the opportunity to impose control on physician behavior by forcing ordering according to "policies." For example, the pharmacy may wish to decrease the demand for an expensive antibiotic. The approach can be to present all ordering of that antibiotic on-line or provide a long list of warning screens before the order can be completed, in the hopes of discouraging the request for that medication. Alternatively, the PCIS can be designed to educate the ordering physician with a few important bits of information *before* the order is completed, e.g., the list of antibiotics that the patient's infection is sensitive to *and* the relative costs of those antibiotics. Additionally, warnings on side effects of medications should be easily available to the clinician before he or she finishes an order, particularly when there are interactions between a drug and the patient's other medications.

Integrated results reporting is an essential component of a PCIS. The process of patient care obviously has the patient as its central focus. Unfortunately, in the process of caring for patients in today's hospitals, the information collected on patients is compartmentalized in many different areas. For example, pathology information in the pathology system, pharmacy information in the pharmacy department with an additional copy in the nursing area, etc. Because the clinician must have all of the important data on a patient to make the best informed decisions, we turn a fragmented, decentralized body of data into a patient-centered, integrated information resource for it to be most useful. The PCIS must be tightly integrated with all information resources in the hospital containing all elements of the patient's data.

In the final analysis, the effectiveness of a PCIS can be directly related to the robustness of its communications and patient scheduling capabilities. In the process of patient care, many individuals require notification, reminders, and special clinical information to deliver that care successfully. For example, to accomplish a cardiac catheterization, there must be coordination and communication among nursing, radiology, cardiology, and cardiac surgery. Additionally, laboratory, dietary, housekeeping, and other services must be aware of the scheduled test to avoid sending lab technicians to an empty room, feeding the patient just before the test, etc. Because of the complexity and number of tests on each patient, each day, it often falls on nursing to maintain the flow of patients and information to complete the day's tasks. Therefore, the PCIS must comprehensively support the communication "chain of command, so that care is delivered to the patient in the most effective and efficient manner possible. From the physician's standpoint, the communications capabilities of the PCIS should also include warning of test preparation interactions (e.g., performing the colonoscopy prior to the barium enema) and the ability for the attending physician to request consultation on-line and review results on-line. Finally, the need for PCIS communications links extends to physicians' offices, freestanding medical clinics, and surgical centers. With these communications and long-term patient records, the PCIS acts as the central nervous system of the patient's medical information, allowing more effective coordination and interaction among all those responsible for the patient's care.

Physician reminders, a unique benefit of PCIS, have only rarely been fully utilized. At the Latter Day Saints Hospital in Salt Lake City, Utah, there is an information HELP system[2] that stands as the best example of an information system integrated with a system of clinical reminders. Most of our quality assurance systems in medicine are retrospective. We develop criteria for clinical performances and then apply them to actual experience in selected areas of our hospitals and cite exceptions. We then notify physicians responsible for those exceptions with the hope that this influence will improve the outcome of the next group of patients those doctors care for. However, we usually do nothing to help influence clinicians' decisions *before* the very next occurrence of the quality issue. For example, many hospitals (and the Joint Commission on Accreditation of Healthcare Organizations) have been concerned about the use of blood products in obstetrical patients. Criteria have been determined for appropriate use of blood in these patients and circulated to medical staffs. QA departments monitor the use of blood products from these areas and, when excessive use is identified, contact the responsible physicians to help explain the reasons for the occurrence. If this same information was consistently presented to clinicians in the same pathways used to order blood products, we would have a unique opportunity to *prospectively* influence clinicians' decision and make them aware that their performance is considered an important quality of care issue. The emphasis would be effectively shifted from a retrospective punitive process to a prospective, "let me help you make the best decision" process. The implications are obvious, both for physician acceptance and for effect on the next patient's outcome.

A patient's health care does not begin and end with a hospitalization, an outpatient clinic visit, or a consultation with a physician. The health care of a patient is a compendium of all health care encounters for the life of the patient. Therefore, patient care information systems must be capable of collecting, storing, and effectively presenting information for the entire life span of the individual patient. Until recently, the computing power and storage capability to meet this need were not available. Today, however, the technology is available to meet this challenge effectively. What remains is the continued design and development of information systems to support the clinical needs of presenting data successfully. For example, during clinical decision making, the physician would have to query this long-term patient database across all episodes of care in health care settings. In a long-term outpatient clinic, (e.g., an internal medicine health maintenance clinic), information would be sought specific to that clinic for each and every encounter that patient had with that clinic. Tabular, graphic, and summary information presentation tools must continue to be developed to allow clinicians to make successful use of the large volumes of clinical information that we need to review on our patients and convert that data into real medical information.

Concurrent medical education has been recognized for many years as the most effective means of educating medical students and residents. Yet, because of the high cost of manpower and time, it is all too rare in most medical school curricula. The bedside experience with a learned clinician at the time of first patient interview is often an experience that is relished and remembered for many years by physicians. A PCIS cannot replace these experiences, but it can provide a unique opportunity to deliver important education information in context with the work-up and evaluation of a patient, both to the physician in training and the experienced clinician. Over the past 10 years, there has been a remarkable surge of popularity of on-line medical literature retrieval (i.e., MEDLINE).[3] The next level of clinical education is the integration of the medical literature into the day-to-day practice of clinical decision making, orders, and results. To accomplish this goal, PCIS must contain a structure of identifying active patient problems so that subsystems can retrieve and present relevant clinical literature for the physician's review. Clinical departments also have an opportunity to educate physicians through user-selectable medical information supplements to the clinical service part of their portion of the PCIS. For example, while ordering medications from the pharmacy, the physician may also review that section of the on-line PDR and drug interaction database for more detail on drug metabolism and actions. In this way, the less familiar medications and treatments can be successfully introduced to the medical staff in a consistent and predictable manner.

The PCIS, with its longitudinal record of clinical information and rich database of patient information, is the ideal driving system for a clinical research information system. Although the speed and operational requirements of a research database may be different from a PCIS, the important barrier to collecting complete clinical information for clinical research and outcomes study *is* the front end of the process: the interaction at the time of care delivery that the PCIS embodies. With this connection between a relational research database and a PCIS, clinicians are able to evaluate, with security safeguards, all of the important clinical experience with a particular medical system. Implications for using the experience of a medical center for determining the most efficient and effective management strategies are·extremely important, especially in the current climate of out-of-control health care costs.

There several major directions patient care information systems will be taking in the future:

- Improvement in information presentation (the physician/executive information system.

- Multimedia integration completing the electronic medical record.

- Improvement in the person-machine interface.

As patient care information systems become more and more comprehensive repositories of a patient's clinical record, there will be more data to present to the clinician for review and decision making. Navigating this sea of information is no small task and will require innovative strategies of presenting clinical data to allow clinicians to convert it into information. Several probable trends include GUI, EIS, and DSS.

GUI (graphic user interface) provides the opportunity of presenting familiar objects to the user in the course of using the PCIS. This may accomplish several goals: faster training in the use of the PCIS, more rapid navigation through the wealth of patient data in the PCIS because all areas of the system operate in a similar and familiar manner, and more intimate integration of the PCIS into the clinician's daily practice. This last goal bears some explanation. The "heads up display" is today's fighter pilot's best instrument for keeping track of the thousands of bits of information that he or she must process while trying to use a modern jet aircraft. This device, built as part of the pilot's helmet, provides iconic displays of the status of vital fighter systems using motion and color to alert the pilot to the stable, caution, or urgent status of these systems. A simple glance over these displays provides all the important information needed. When the PCIS contains the vital patient information, is interfaced to patient monitoring devices, and is more portable and "personal" in the future, these graphic displays will be invaluable to alert the busy clinician to time-critical information and allow review of less urgent data during standard rounding hours. In this way, the busy clinician of the future will have an electronic link, far more sophisticated than today's "beepers," containing prioritized, vital information necessary to maintain complete control over his or her practice. Because this information instrument will be a PCIS, the clinician will be able to receive data and transmit instructions and orders using a single device, thereby saving time and improving accuracy and quality of care.

EIS (executive information systems) are currently available information systems that allow graphical summarization of vast amounts of business information for the busy executive and provide the ability to obtain more detailed data as needed. The parallel between this capability, and the requirement of the busy clinician to successfully use the large amount of data available in a PCIS, are quite similar and have similar time constraints. The same structure that creates today's EIS will be used in the PCIS of the future to allow the clinician to more effectively navigate the longitudinal database to the precise patient information he or she is after. One feature of the EIS that will be most useful for the clinician is "drill down," which allows the user to select a bit of summary information, request the data behind that information, request the data detail behind that, etc. For example, the clinician may select a problem such as asthma. He is then presented with the results of pulmonary function tests and a pulmonary consultant report that led to the diagnosis. He can request the display of each individual episode of care that involved that diagnosis and the outcomes of therapy. This capability would be most helpful to the clinician *across* patients. For example, the same clinician may wish to compare how he has done in treating asthma compared to his colleagues. He wishes to look at length of hospitalizations of asthmatics and how often his patients return to the hospital as compared with a blinded listing of his colleagues' performance, and perhaps even with national standards.

DSS (decision support software) will allow the PCIS of the future to recommend diagnostic and therapeutic strategies to the clinician on the basis of analysis of the large amount of patient-specific information available in the longitudinal database, as well as of clinical algorithms developed by local or national "expert" groups. This case management facility will allow faster conversion of the sea of clinical data available on a patient into real information. Serious concerns have been raised in this regard concerning the liability of software authors for incorrect diagnosis or treatment. Obviously, the current state of medical litigation would require significant change before such systems could be widely implemented. Nevertheless, in response to the current health care crisis, many hospitals are developing their own practice guidelines for specialty-expensive or high-risk procedures. With the PCIS of the future, such guidelines could be automatically incorporated into *all* clinicians' daily routines, thereby, improving the *average* clinical performance for an entire medical community.

With current advances in multimedia presentation via computer, including voice, pictures, and video, the PCIS of the future will take advantage of this technology to present an electronic medical record far more complete than the current paper record. For example, the review of the ECG will be possible directly from the display of the report of the test by clicking on the ECG icon. The chest x-ray, CT, and MRI images will be displayable likewise on the same terminal screen that permits report review and ordering. The multimedia PCIS will allow voice mail on-line that really *is* the face and voice of the consultant you've asked to give you information on this patient. Real-time, on-line communication using video and voice is likewise possible via remote network connections allowing teleconferencing and teleconsultation, avoiding the need to transfer patient and records miles away to specialized, medical centers.

To be successful in the future, the PCIS must be available to clinicians in a better match between person and machine. The current terminal requires a break in workflow—sitting down and using a keyboard, lightpen, mouse, or some other device to communicate through the system. The lackluster acceptance of bedside terminals, except in critical care areas, has taught us that, to be effective, computer devices need to be where the action is. Therefore, demands on technology will produce a new generation of portable, wireless devices that begin where the beeper systems left off. They will be full-function connections to the PCIS—light (containing a variety of input and output choices), voice, tablet, keyboard, etc.—and will be kept *with* the clinician as the devices alert the user to important information that has been received and requires urgent action. Likewise, these portable devices will allow two-way communication with other clinicians, replacing the endless "telephone tag" so common today. As all clinicians will need a personal information device to be in close communication, these information instruments will finally be as much a part of the physicians "little black bag" as is the stethoscope. It is at this stage of development that the PCIS and computers in general will achieve the ultimate transition from foreign devices to information appliances.

## Research

A significant portion of research is data collection, data reduction, and analysis. While it is extremely important to define these steps correctly, the actual accomplishment can be very laborious and repetitious. It was recognized very early on that the coming of age of computers could free the researcher from these tasks.

In the 1960s and 1970s, data were stored in mainframe computers, and programmers were required to access data and write analysis programs.[4,5] Process control systems were expensive and very difficult to program. In 1979, an early process control computer was programmed to run two automated blood analyzers in the pathology laboratories at University Hospital at Stony Brook. The programming was complex and difficult and required many hours of highly specialized programming. When changes had to be made after the original programmer left, they were difficult to accomplish, necessitating a search for new and improved technologies.

Enter the personal computer. The personal computer has changed the way the world perceives and manipulates data. Microchip technology has brought the power of large, mainframe computers to the researcher's desk. In addition to managing clinical and research data on a desktop, personal computer, word processing systems, electronic mail systems, statistical analysis systems, and communications with colleagues all over the world, as well as access to national databases, are now available.

As early as 1983, Joseph G. Sladen, MD, presented a paper to the 70th Annual Meeting of the North Pacific Surgical Association[6] describing the use of a personal computer to define and manage databases. Dr. Sladen states that "the personal computer gives direct contact with your data, and allows you to see your files and develop your ideas. It is the method of the future today." The relative simplicity of use allowed the researcher to access and manipulate the data directly, without the requirement of a programmer as an intermediary. Dr. Sladen describes the tools he used to analyze his data, develop graphic representations of the data, and then create slides to be used in presentation of his findings. In addition, standard direct interfaces were developed that allowed personal computers to be directly linked to laboratory equipment. Personal computers can now directly control complex experiments, while simultaneously collecting data.

With the growth of personal computing, the next logical step was to link two or more personal computers so that users could share information and resources. Thus, the need for local area networks (LANs) was created. Today, many departments have internal LANs linking offices and laboratories. The LANs facilitate electronic mail within the department and allow researchers to edit papers and move data between the office and the lab.[7]

The growth of data requirements in research has led to a need for more and more computing capacity. Although there are now exceedingly powerful desktop computers available, more powerful than the mainframes of the early '70s, LANs are frequently tied into departmental minicomputers that may act as file servers for the department (they have more file capacity than the desktop) or as communications routers to tie into other departmental or medical center LANs, or that may handle other departmental computing functions.

D. Preston Flanigan, MD, describes the use of a departmental system that includes access to surgical literature; storage and retrieval of patient registry, laboratory, and research data; generation of reports; statistical analysis of data; and word processing at the University of Illinois College of Medicine.[8] Dr. Flanigan states, "Perhaps the greatest benefit of the system has been the improvement in the quality of our research effort. Research fellows are now encouraged to prepare datasets in the computer before any experimentation. The writing of the statistical programs before experimentation has reduced the amount of retrospective thinking in data analysis. The ability to analyze data without having to re-enter data into separate programs has greatly accelerated the data analysis process."

What about the hospital's mainframe computer? This, too, acts as an extensive source of data for medical center researchers. The mainframe computer can act as a large file server across departmental lines. This gives everyone access to the data they require. The PCIS described above develops significant amounts of data that can be used concurrently in clinical trials, as well as retrospectively for collection, reduction, and analysis of clinical data.

The vascular surgery system described by Dr. Flanigan[8] resides on a mainframe computer. Dr. Flanigan states in his paper that "although the system described within is mainframe-computer based, newer microcomputer operating systems, communications software, and local area networks will allow for the development of similar systems using microcomputer hardware and software."

The combination of individual desktop computing, departmental LANs, and medical center information systems provides a powerful information gathering research team. The need for more and more computing power has driven computing platforms from thousands of instructions per second (KIPS), to millions of instructions per second (MIPS), to billions of mathematical calculations per second (gigaflops). At today's speeds, instructions per second is no longer a valid measurement. We are now approaching the realm of trillions of calculations per second (teraflops). A trillion mathematical instructions is the equivalent of doing in a computer in one second what a person could do entering one calculation per second into a hand-held calculator, 24 hours a day, 365 days a year, for 31,709 years.[9]

There are many cost-effective ways to use computers in today's research environment. Hardware and software improvements are being announced daily. Software is becoming more user-friendly. The researcher can concentrate on doing the research and using the computer as a tool of that research rather than the researcher becoming the tool of the computer. There is less of a requirement for the researcher to become computer literate; computers are becoming more people literate.

## Education

The body of knowledge that medical students must learn increases exponentially each year. The sheer magnitude of the tasks of both teaching and learning this vast body of information in the first two years of medical school suggests that medical schools must provide more student-directed and student-generated learning activities. The movement away from a standard curriculum that requires students to sit through day-long lectures and laboratories in a linear and very structured approach, requiring student recall of isolated facts, to a more participative and guided process reflects the coming of age of multimedia capabilities on computers and the increasing use of interactive computer-aided instruction.

To implement this self-guided learning process, the University of Michigan Medical School has developed "Advanced Tools for Learning Anatomical Structure" (ATLAS plus), an interactive, multimedia, electronic textbook used in the study of anatomical sciences. The software program integrates the use of digitized images, pictures, computer graphics, sound, animations, and textual information to present tutorials on histology (epithelium, connective tissue, bone structure and growth, and muscle), embryology (development of the human face, teratology), and gross anatomy (respiratory system, digestive system, and nervous system).[10]

This process was designed to allow the student to link to sections within the lesson, as well as to other lessons. For example, a student in the bone lesson might want to access information in the connective tissue lesson. A student also has the ability to skip information that is already known. ATLAS plus contains a series of laboratory introductions that are designed to introduce students to the cells and tissues they will be viewing during the laboratory session.

Digitized images are displayed, accompanied by text describing important tissues and structures. First-time users are encouraged to follow the lessons systematically to become familiar with the program's flow. In subsequent uses of the laboratory introductions, students may simply review images, changing the flow to suit individual needs.

The use of programs such as ATLAS plus in schools of medicine will not only provide medical students with a powerful learning tool that meets their current need to acquire significant volumes of information, but it will focus on the need to teach medical students to be lifelong learners as well.

Another approach to computer-aided medical education is the use of ILIAD, a system that can operate as an expert medical system and as a support to teaching. There has been widespread resistance to the use of expert medical systems as clinical consultants. These same systems, when used in simulation mode, can generate an inexhaustible supply of simulated cases and can direct the development of questioning and reasoning skills much as an expert teacher would.[11]

A student would use ILIAD by beginning with a chief complaint. The student then asks questions about the patient's condition, requests results from the physical examination, and orders diagnostic studies. The student can then develop a diagnosis. ILIAD will respond to the diagnosis with suggestions on narrowing it down.

In a paper presented at the thirteenth annual "Symposium on Computer Applications in Medical Care," November 5-8, 1989, the Department of Medical Informatics of the University of Utah School of Medicine concluded that the ILIAD simulator can improve medical student problem solving skills. The conclusion was based on a study in which all third-year medical students received standardized cases generated on the simulator. The students attempted to identify the diagnoses, presented questions to the simulator, and received answers about the simulated findings. The task of the students was to continue selecting findings until they could make a diagnosis with enough confidence that they would be willing to begin treatment of the patient.

In this very carefully controlled environment, the researchers concluded that students perform better at the end of their clerkship experience than at the beginning of the rotation. "In particular, students were able to pursue history findings that have greater information value at the end of their rotation than they could at the beginning."[11]

A well-defined PCIS also adds to the learning experience. For example, when the PCIS recommends generic drugs or lists the hospital's P&T requirements for a certain drug therapy before that drug can be ordered, that is a learning opportunity. When the PCIS presents the criteria for ordering specific diagnostic modalities, that presents a learning opportunity. In effect, there is a commonality between the system for implementing clinical care and teaching students how to use that care.

# Conclusion

The tradition of independence of thought and action in the academic medical school environment has created a very nourishing environment for the creative development of new ideas and processes. Individual creativity is the cornerstone upon which new ideas are born. The academic health center must continue to nourish this environment to challenge the frontiers of medical knowledge.

There has been a realization that recent reductions in reimbursement formulas and in the availability of research funds must lead to the pooling of common interests. Shared use of information systems facilitates the integration of the care providing, research, and teaching missions of the academic health center. There is continuous learning and teaching while providing care. The boundaries among the missions are almost indistinguishable.

Although there are many specialized programs and systems that support the missions, the cornerstone, upon which all are built, should be the patient care information system. PCIS provides the information for clinical decision making, the extracts for research, and a powerful teaching tool.

The integration of the medical center's information into a readily accessible, integrated repository is very exciting. The use of the information that can be accessed under an integrated schema is limited only to the imaginations of the people who need that access. The future is indeed bright for those who have the desire to reach out for it.

# References

1   Gall, J., and others. "Demonstration and Evaluation of a Total Hospital Information System." NCHSR Research Summary Series, U.S. Department of Health Education and Welfare Public Health Service, Health Resources Administration, HRA77-3188.

2   Gardner, R., and others. "Computer-Critiqued Blood Ordering Using the HELP System." *Computers and Biomedical Research* 23(6):514-28, Dec. 1990.

3   Bachrach, C., and Charen, T. "Selection of MEDLINE Contents, the Development of Its Thesaurus, and the Indexing Process." *Medical Informatics* (London) 3(3):237-54, Sept. 1978.

4   Litherland, H. "Impact of Computer Technology on Analysis of Results of Peripheral Arterial Operations." *American Surgery* 38(9):477-80, Sept. 1972.

5   Cameron, A. "The Value of Gastroscopy in Clinical Diagnosis, A Computer Aided Study." *Mayo Clinic Proceedings* 52(12):806-8, Dec. 1977.

6   Sladen, J. "The Personal Computer as a Clinical Research and Teaching Tool." *American Journal of Surgery* 147(5):654-9, May 1984.

7   Ziegler, K. *Distributed Computing and the Mainframe.* New York, N.Y.: John Wiley & Sons, 1991.

8   Flanigan, D. "Computerization of Academic Vascular Surgery." *Surgery* 106(5):911-9, Nov. 1989.

9   "Special Report: Where No Computer Has Gone Before." *Business Week*, Nov. 25, 1991.

10  Love, S., and others. "Design Techniques for Ensuring Structure and Flexibility in a Hypermedia Environment." *Multimedia Review* 2(2):34-43, Summer 1991.

11  Warner, H. "ILIAD: A Diagnostic Consultant and Patient Stimulator." Expert System." *MD Computing* 8(1):46-53, Jan. 1991.

*Paul R. Vegoda is Chief Information Officer and William F. Bria, MD, is Medical Director, Clinical Information Systems and Critical Care Medicine Unit, University of Michigan Hospitals, Ann Arbor, Mich.*

# Chapter 13

# Training Medical Managers at the Academic Health Center

*by Judith Cooksey, MD, MPH, and Roger Hand, MD*

## Clinicians as Managers

Since the mid-1960s, with the introduction of Medicaid and Medicare, the U.S. health care system has grown increasingly complex. Indeed, in the 1980s, the proliferation of multiple delivery models, financing methods, and regulatory systems became so great that many clinicians, in medicine, nursing, pharmacy and other allied health professions, found themselves overwhelmed by the changes. Some, in leadership positions in health care organizations, found themselves practicing health care management. Most of these managers got to their positions by virtue of seniority or their excellence as clinicians rather than expertise or training in management. They learned their jobs on the job. As with all clinical specialties, there has been an evolution, and it is no longer acceptable simply to declare one's self an expert in medical management and then go out to practice it. Formal or informal training is required. Academic health centers have a clear responsibility for providing this training.

Only a minority of physicians currently holding management positions have had this training. A 1986 study of more than 14,000 physicians whose primary responsibility was administration found that less than 13 percent had a management master's degree. Ten percent held degrees in public health, with the remainder in business administration and management.[1] A more recent study of 1,200 hospital-based members of the American College of Physician Executives found that 16 percent had a master's degree and 10 percent were working on a degree.[2]

While few physician managers possess a degree in a management discipline, many have received some training through continuing education courses. Some professional schools, such as pharmacy and nursing, have offered management courses within their undergraduate curricula and have developed administration and management programs leading to a master's degrees in management within their schools. Medical schools have lagged behind in this area until recently.

The venue for much of the management training for clinicians is the academic health center. As the health center is frequently located within a university, the faculty and course offerings from nonhealth professional colleges can be utilized. In this chapter, we review degree and nondegree programs in clinical management and offer suggestions for education and training.

## Management Models in Academic Health Centers

Within an academic health center, many management models exist, with varying administrative or management roles for clinicians. From the medical school vantage, Petersdorf has described four key leadership positions: the vice president for health services, the dean of medicine, department heads, and the hospital director.[3] Each has a critical role in governance and administration and important interactive responsibilities. In an analysis of leadership and management within academic health centers, Wilson and McLaughlin identified several critical responsibilities for department heads.[4] The head manages the department, makes decisions about resource allocation, resolves personnel issues, recruits faculty, and carries out strategic planning. He or she also serves as an advocate and representative for the department to internal and external groups and shares responsibility in overall management and long-term well-being of the institution (medical school or medical center).

Within departments, management of clinical practice requires oversight and planning in both the medical and business arenas. Although most practices have business managers, the faculty member responsible for the practice requires an understanding of personnel and staffing, office management, quality assurance, patient recruitment, marketing, billing, and reimbursement issues. As medical school and health center budgets become more dependent on practice-generated revenues, the demands for practice management expertise are increasing.

Another common management model within a university, college, or hospital is the committee chairmanship. While many complain of the time demands and frustrations of committee work, committees serve important functions for organizations, ranging from recruitment (search committees and resident committees), monitoring and oversight, crisis intervention (ad hoc groups to address a specific problem), new program development, and long-term planning. Management in these settings requires skill in interpersonal and group interactions, understanding of institutional organization and functions, and efficiency in carrying out delegated tasks.

## Concerns about Management Responsibilities

Despite the many opportunities for faculty to become involved with management, there is often a reluctance to take on this responsibility. Some of the concerns are understandable, such as the time involved, adding one more demand to a full plate of clinical, teaching, and research demands; lack of interest; frustrations with bureaucracy; and lack of experience. However, there may be other less recognized reasons for avoiding management responsibilities. Physicians may find it difficult to extend their professional domain beyond their area of training and expertise. The traditional medical training model, which requires a lengthy apprenticeship before assuming leadership responsibility, contrasts with real-life experiences. Often, the opportunity to take on a management role or responsibility must be seized without a long preparation time.

Many management settings require the administrative leader to function through negotiation, sharing of power, and reliance on nonphysicians for expertise. These differ from clinical settings, which are structurally hierarchical, with physician dominance. One may have to learn about new areas not covered in prior training or work experiences. Decision making must take into account the complexities of regulation, finance, and personnel issues. Problem solving does not easily allow application of the scientific method, and solutions often cannot be tested before they must be applied.

Despite these concerns, there are positive aspects of participating in health care management. Increasingly, decisions about health care are made by lay managers, economists, and policy analysts, with only limited input from clinicians. Hillman and his colleagues have made an elegant argument that there is a critical role for properly trained physician executives to face the challenge of managing the medical-industrial complex and designing rational programs for health care delivery.[3] Many physicians who have chosen careers in administration cite as reasons their desire to have a broad impact on and to improve the quality of health care.[1]

## Topics for Training Programs

A decade ago, medical management was defined as quality assurance, utilization review, and risk management. These three areas still form the "clinical" core of medical management. However, most clinicians would find themselves at a disadvantage in working with administrators if this was the limit of their knowledge. A broader exposure is necessary for education and training programs. An in-depth understanding of the health care delivery system is critical. This includes the environmental factors affecting the system, such as epidemiology, finance systems, and regulatory issues. Medical statistics, medical information systems, and health care policy should also be offered. Traditional management topics should be covered, if possible, from the perspective of health care organizations. These include organizational structure and theory; management and leadership tools, such as decision making, communication, and change and conflict management; and management processes, such as planning, financial control, human resource management, and control and evaluation (including traditional quality assurance, utilization review, and risk management). Finally, the prospective medical manager should have exposure to medical policy and power to include some appreciation of the role of government, market forces, professional organizations, and labor in the health care system.

## Training Program Models

Clinicians considering training in management have a broad range of options. While many skills can be acquired through on-the-job experiences, organized learning programs have advantages and are increasingly recognized as valued prerequisites for management positions. Training programs can be considered in two general categories: nondegree and formal degree programs. Nondegree programs, such as seminars, workshops, fellowships, peer learning experiences, and mentorship programs cover many of the topics discussed above. Degree programs, usually master's level, are offered in business, health administration, public health, and related areas. There are a small but growing number of degree programs that have been developed specifically for clinicians.

Workshops and seminars are probably the most common choice for a training experience. These are offered by professional associations, universities, and private sector accounting, management, or consulting firms and cover topics in general management or health-related issues. They are usually of short duration (a few hours to several days) and tend to address current issues. They offer a problem-solving and skills-building approach rather than theoretical or in-depth analysis.

Health management professional associations seek to develop programs that meet the needs of their membership. For example, the American College of Physician Executives offers a three-part series of Physician in Management

Seminars. Each seminar lasts five days and covers topics of interest to physicians (health systems organization, economics of health care, regulation, and competition) as well as general management issues (planning, implementing change, staff issues, and productivity).[6] Membership in a professional management association also provides an opportunity to meet colleagues who share interests and to establish a professional identity affiliated with management. The informal exchange of experiences with members can provide a peer learning experience and a useful network of associates.

Another important training model that occurs in fields as diverse as business, academics, and research and can be critical to career development is the mentorship model. By its nature, this model requires special circumstances and commitment and is an individualized experience. In academic health centers, mentoring is a strong element of clinical and research training programs. Formal mentorship programs in administration are uncommon; however, an interesting model has been developed by the Association of Academic Health Centers. Its Leadership Diversity Program was started in 1991 and provides an opportunity for senior faculty members to work with leaders of health science centers and the Washington-based association. The program hopes to provide women and minority faculty with a series of experiences that will prepare them for leadership positions in academic health centers.[7]

Another training model that offers an intense, individualized experience is the professional fellowship. These are select and often prestigious awards that may involve up to a year of work and study. The Robert Wood Johnson Health Policy Fellowship is offered to mid-career faculty from academic health professions who wish to study health policy and take on leadership roles in health-related areas. This program admits six fellows to a year-long experience in Washington, with assignments to key congressional offices. Although the focus in on health policy, graduates often assume key leadership positions in universities, government, and the private sector.[8]

Several universities have implemented faculty development training programs to enhance teaching, clinical practice, or management skills. These programs usually last one to four weeks and provide an intensive group learning experience guided by senior faculty. A variant of this model aimed at university-based faculty and staff in mid-level management positions is offered by Harvard University School of Education. The Management Development Program uses the case method of study, formal lectures, and small group discussions to cover university management and leadership issues, including those related to academic health centers.[9]

The decision to enter a degree program usually reflects a commitment to a more in-depth study of management and its application. It is often tied to a career shift or expectation.[10] Degree programs require a substantial commitment of time, money, energy, and often travel over a one- or two-year period. University-based programs are available in business administration, health administration, public health, public administration, policy analysis, and management. Many offer special executive programs designed for individuals at mid-career that involve considerably less on-campus time. They offer an attractive alternative for those planning to continue working while pursing a degree. The cost of executive programs generally runs $18,000 to $20,000 for the two-year program.

Northwestern University offers an executive program in general management through the Kellogg Graduate School of Management that leads to a master's of management degree. The Executive Master's Program is aimed at mid-career executives, including health professionals, and is conducted over two years through full-day lecture/seminars held on alternate Fridays and Saturdays on campus. The curriculum includes 12 six-week modules covering contemporary management issues. Students work in study groups that generally meet at least once a week; the groups form a critical part of the learning experience.[11]

A health-focused executive program is offered by the University of Colorado Graduate School of Business Administration. Approximately one-third of the class members are physicians, another third are clinicians from nursing and allied health professions, and the final third are nonclinical managers.[12] The program is decentralized, in that students spend only 10 weeks of a two-year period on campus (after an orientation, 2 weeks every 6 months). The program relies heavily on the microcomputer as an educational medium for computer conferencing and on electronic seminars, lectures, discussions, mail, and homework evaluation. Course work covers general management and health-related issues and leads to a master's of science in health administration degree.

The University of Wisconsin-Madison offers master's of science degrees in administrative medicine in cooperation with the American College of Physician Executives. This program, which began in 1979, was the first in the country dedicated to training clinician-executives and to linking clinical perspectives with health care administration.[13] Currently, the program recruits physicians and nurses who have administrative responsibilities or are planning a career change into management. The nonresident program requires a 22-month study period of four semesters, including six 10-day sessions on campus. Courses are offered in business and management fundamentals and medical management applications.

A growing number of pharmacy and nursing schools offer programs with business schools that lead to combined master's degrees in the primary health discipline and in business administration. For example, the University of Illinois College of Nursing offers a combined MSN/MBA program with the College of Business Administration. The 24-month program includes core courses in business administration and nursing administration and a practicum experience. Graduates plan careers in nursing and health care administration.[14]

Schools of medicine and dentistry have offered joint programs for a combined MD or DDS and MPH degree. Some medical schools offer public health degree programs within their curricula; other rely on university-affiliated schools of public health. Some health professional schools have developed joint programs with business schools leading to an MBA degree. For example, the Wharton School at the University of Pennsylvania offers students in medicine and dental medicine combined MD/MBA and DMD/MBA degrees.[15] Students apply to each program separately and usually require an additional 18 months to complete the combined programs.

## Training Opportunities within an Academic Health Center

Although formal degree programs in management offer the most rigorous training to health care professionals interested in management, there is the need for academic health centers to offer education in management at other levels. Most health professionals who practice patient care devote some time to management activities. Organized medicine today requires clinicians to take part in quality assurance and utilization review activities, to be involved in business and marketing projects for their hospitals or group practices, to organize and lead other clinicians for the efficient and efficacious delivery of health care, and to be aware of changing trends in the health care field.

Academic health centers, by virtue of their educational mission, have a special opportunity to train professionals in management, and many do. The lead here has been taken by schools of nursing and pharmacy, many of which have academic departments of administration.

Medical schools, in contrast, have lagged behind. Formal courses in practice management are unusual, although prospective employers of physicians, such as HMOs, regard such education as important,[16] and physicians themselves recognize the need for it.[17] As recently as the mid-1970s, less than 25 percent of medical schools offered any instruction in quality assurance and less than 10 percent had courses.[18,19] By 1989, 105 of 127 medical schools surveyed by the American Medical Association offered some instruction in quality assurance and utilization review, but few provided more than a handful of hours.[20] According to a more recent survey, 27 percent of 98 responding medical schools offered a course or related program in quality assurance, compared to 61 percent of 69 degree programs in health administration.[21] In a questionnaire asking medical schools whether they taught the broader topic of health care delivery and finance, 75 percent of responders did, but less than 25 percent offered it as a required course or had more than 20 hours of instruction in the topic.[22] In the most recent AMA survey,[23] of 124 responding medical schools, some hours were devoted to health care systems in 101, to medical informatics in 48, to practice management in 52, to technology assessment in 37, and to utilization review and quality assurance in 70.

Postgraduate training in medical management is now available through a limited number of fellowships and residency programs. Fellowships are aimed at future academic physicians who have completed a residency in a clinical discipline. They are offered in medical informatics, medical decision making, and health care policy. The first formal residency in quality assurance and utilization review was started at Hershey Medical College in the mid-1980s,[24] and several others have come into existence since then.[25] Presently, there are no more than four throughout the country.[26] These programs, in addition to teaching quality assurance and utilization review, provide instruction in organizational analysis and development and in medical informatics.[27] There have been suggestions for more extensive development of quality assurance programs at academic centers that would be the focus for research and teaching up through the fellowship level.[28]

Board certification is now available to physicians in medical management[29] and in quality assurance and utilization review.[30] Neither board has yet been recognized as a medical specialty by the American Board of Medical Specialties. Eligibility is determined by postgraduate training through a relevant master's degree program or continuing medical education experience.

Because all health professionals can anticipate involvement in medical management during their careers, academic health centers have a responsibility for providing some training to all their students, be they in medicine, nursing, dentistry, pharmacy or the allied health professions. Because medical schools have lagged behind in this area and because there is a perceived need for medical education reform to make it more relevant,[31] the time may be propitious to increase the prominence of management subjects in medical school curricula.

## Management Training in Undergraduate and Graduate Medical Education

Principles and applications of medical management can be taught at three levels of medical education: preclinical years, clinical years, and residency. Training should be incremental and should reinforce concepts through clinical applications, as the traditional medical training model does. For example, the important concepts of a clinical condition are taught first through the basic sciences. Then, in the clinical years, students learn about diagnosis and management through patient contact and faculty-guided correlation of the clinical and basic science aspects of cases. In the graduate years, the resident will manage cases with increasing independence, applying knowledge from the basic and clinical sciences. Medical management should be taught in the same way: basic concepts, clinical applications, and supervised practice. We will describe a model curriculum for medical management. Although designed for medical students, with modification it can be used for students in any of the health professions.

The "basic science" of medical management is the structure and function of the health care delivery system. Beginning students may have some familiarity with it through personal experiences and prior education. The subject can be introduced in the first year and can offer a welcome respite from the rigors of anatomy and biochemistry. It can easily be taught in small group discussions, although some of the material lends itself to lecture format. The topics should include health problems of the nation—the distribution of major diseases; the national costs of medical care; the problems of special populations, such as children and the elderly; inequities in access to health care; the influence of technology, and important trends, such as the growth of ambulatory care. The geographic and specialty distribution of health workers and the changing roles of providers are also important topics. Issues affecting health care delivery, such as managed care, health insurance and reimbursement systems, regulatory agencies, medical malpractice, health care policy, and legislation should also be discussed.

Approximately 10 hours of instruction will cover these subjects in sufficient detail to give students background for further readings on their own. A related and important topic that should be introduced in the first year is medical informatics, which should be given in sufficient detail to allow students to take full advantage of a medical library. An interesting elective that can be introduced at this point is comparative health care systems.

Later in the preclinical years, students can be introduced to medical outcomes research, medical quality and quality assurance, utilization and risk management, and medical decision making. Again, these subjects lend themselves to small group discussions and can be introduced in 10 hours of instruction. They are best taught after students have had some instruction in statistics and epidemiology.

In the 1970s, there were several experimental programs to teach quality assurance and peer review techniques to clinical medical students.[32,33] They were based on retrospective chart audits, which was the system for quality assessment at that time. In a more up-to-date program for clinical students, relevant topics can be integrated into traditional clerkship teaching rounds, such as hospital rounds and morning report, clinic staff meetings, and other patient care or specialty conferences. The focus should be on relating the topics to individual cases. Discussion of access to needed health care and organization of health services can be worked into presentations of individual cases without detracting from traditional discussions of patient management.

Students should also be introduced to programs in quality assurance and utilization review as practiced at the medical center. An orientation and visit to the medical records department and the office of medical information systems can also be useful as part of the clinical teaching programs.

Clinical training programs that use multiple sites for ambulatory training should expose students to management issues involved with differing models of ambulatory practice. These issues may differ in focus, depending on the practice model (individual, group, university-based) and the clientele served. This will provide first-hand knowledge of management issues and challenges associated with the ambulatory practice of medicine.

In the fourth year, faculty can offer electives in any of the subjects covered in the first three years. If there is an ongoing research program in any of the areas, such as outcomes research or technology assessment, an elective experience could be offered to encourage a more in-depth study of the topic.

There have been suggestions that quality assurance techniques can be used to teach residents, particularly on matters of cost containment.[34,35] There are institutions that have introduced such audits as teaching tools in psychiatry,[36] internal medicine,[37] and pediatrics[38] with some effectiveness. However, the method used was retrospective chart review. A more relevant program for residents would be a continuation of that taught to clinical medical students but at a more sophisticated level. Quality assurance and utilization review professionals can meet and orient residents and physicians with an overview of their activities. Attendings should make these topics part of their teaching rounds. In a block rotation in ambulatory care or in an appropriate clinical elective, residents can be given a series of seminars covering management topics. During the same rotation, residents might observe or take part in the utilization review discussions with physician advisors as attendings. Medical director rounds, information systems rounds, and finance rounds can be interesting topics for conferences. Grand rounds should occasionally be devoted to a topic in medical management, and guest speakers may be invited to participate in presentations.

Toward the end of the residency years, special seminars should be offered on practice management. This is best taught in a seminar setting, with a planned series of two- to three-hour sessions using speakers involved in practice management. The instruction should be specific for the specialty but should also include a review of the characteristics of the health care system and important trends and policy issues for the short and mid-term.

As with any teaching at the residency level, the interests and expertise of the attending faculty will help determine the exposure of residents to a particular topic. However, if a subject such as medical management is felt to be important, leadership and direction by the department chair and the program director will ensure that it is appropriately covered.

## Conclusions

Management is a late bloomer in the field of health professional education. A generation ago, medical educators gave little attention to the subject. Today, with the increasing complexity and costs of health care systems, there is a need for a cadre of clinicians who can work side-by-side with health care administrators in the field of medical management. The academic health center can and should train this cadre.

# References

1. Kindig, D., and Lostiri, S. "Administrative Medicine: A New Medical Specialty." *Health Affairs* 5(4):46-56, Winter 1986.

2. Kindig, D., and others. "Career Paths of Physician Executives." *Health Care Management Review* 16(4):11-9, Fall 1991.

3. Petersdorf, R., and Wilson, M. "The Four Horseman of the Apocalypse. Study of Academic Medical Center Governance." *JAMA* 247(8):1153-61, Feb. 26, 1982.

4. Wilson, M., and McLaughlin, C. *Leadership and Management in Academic Medicine.* San Francisco, Calif.: Jossey-Bass, 1984, Chapter 2.

5. Hillman, A., and others. Managing the Medical-Industrial Complex." *New England Journal of Medicine* 315(8):511-3, Aug.21, 1986.

6. Personal communication. American College of Physician Executives, 1992.

7. Personal communication, Association of Academic Health Centers, Proposal for a Leadership Program in Academic Health Centers, 1990.

8. Personal communication. Robert Wood Johnson Foundation, 1992.

9. Personal communication. Harvard University School of Education, 1992.

10. Kindig, D., and Sanborn, A. "Is There a Master's Degree in Your Future." *Physician Executive* 15(1):15-8, Jan.-Feb. 1989.

11. Personal communication. Northwestern University Kellogg Graduate School of Management, 1992.

12. Neumann, B. "Structure and Advantages of a Distributed Educational Model for Health Care Managers." *Journal of Health Administration Education* 7(4):711-22, Fall 1989.

13. Detmer, D., and Noren, J. "An Administrative Medicine Program for Clinician-Executives." *Journal of Medical Education* 56(8):640-45, Aug. 1981.

14. Personal communication. University of Illinois College of Nursing, 1992.

15. Kissick, W. "Health Care Management According to Ben Franklin." *Journal of Health Administration Education* 7(4):723-37, Fall 1989.

16. Jacobs, M., and Mott, P. "Physician Characteristics and Training Emphasis Considered Desirable by Leaders of HMOs." *Journal of Medical Education* 62(9):725-731, Sept. 1987.

17. Hoefflinger-Taft, S., and Pelikan, J. "Clinic Management Teams: Integrators of Professional Service and Environmental Change." *Health Care Management Review* 15(2):67-79, Spring 1990.

18. Kane, R., and Hogben, M. "Teaching Quality of Care Assessment to Medical Students." *Journal of Medical Education* 49(8):778-80, Aug. 1974.

19. Carroll, J., and Becker, S. "The Paucity of Course Work in Medical Care Evaluation." *Journal of Medical Education* 50(1):31-7, Jan. 1975.

20. Jonas, H., and others. "Undergraduate Medical Education." *JAMA* 264(7):801-9, Aug. 15, 1990.

21. Ackerman, F., and Nash, D. "Teaching the Tenets of Quality: A Survey of Medical Schools and Programs in Health Administration." *QRB* 17(6):200-3, June 1991.

22. Thompson, W., and others. "Survey of Courses Offered in U.S. Medical Schools on Health Care Delivery and Finance." *Journal of Medical Education* 62(9):761-3, Sept. 1987.

23. Personal communication. Barbara Barzanky, American Medical Association, 1992.

24. Zeigenfuss, J. "On the Need for a Physician Residency in Quality Assurance." *Quality Assurance and Utilization Review* 1(4):104-8, Nov. 1986.

25. O'Reilly, R., and Zeigenfuss, J. "A Performance Appraisal System for Quality Assurance and Utilization Review Fellows." *Quality Assurance and Utilization Review* 4(3):64-72, Aug. 1989.

26. Personal communication. Joseph Trautlein, MD, Healthpass PPA, Harrisburg, Pa., 1992.

27. Ziegenfuss, J. "Quality Assurance and Utilization Review Residency Training Program Model." American Board of Quality Assurance and Utilization Review Physicians and Pennsylvania State University at Harrisburg, 1986.

28. Wentzel, R. "The Development of Academic Programs for Quality Assessment." *Archives of Internal Medicine* 151(4):653-4, April 1991.

29. Personal communication, American Board of Medical Management, 1992.

30. Personal communication, American Board of Quality Assurance and Utilization Review Physicians, 1992.

31. Cantor, J., and others. "Medical Educators' View on Medical Education Reform." *JAMA* 265(8):1002-6, Feb, 27, 1991.

32. Garg, M., and others. "Quality in Medical Practice: A Student Program." *Journal of Medical Education* 52(6):514-6, June 1977.

33. Greenbaum, D., and Hoban, J. "Teaching Peer Review at Michigan State University." *Journal of Medical Education* 51(5):392-4, May 1976.

34. Garg, M., and others. "Teaching Students the Relationship between Quality and Cost of Medical Care." *Journal of Medical Education* 50(12, Part 1):1085-91, Dec. 1975.

35. Everett, G. "Quality Assurance and Cost Containment in Teaching Hospitals: Implications for a Period of Economic Restraint." *QRB* 11(2):42-6, Feb. 1985.

36. Awad, A. "Integrating a Clinical Review Process with Postgraduate Training in Clinical Psychopharmacology." *QRB* 13(8):279-82, Aug. 1987.

37. Bouchard, R., and others. "The Impact of a Quality Assurance Program on Postgraduate Training in Internal Medicine." *JAMA* 253(8):1146-50, Feb. 22, 1985.

38. Schor, E. "Teaching Quality Assurance at an HMO." *Journal of Medical Education* 55(2):129-31, Feb. 1980.

*Judith Cooksey, MD, MPH, is Associate Vice Chancellor for Health Services and Roger Hand, MD, is Chief, Section of General Internal Medicine, Department of Medicine, University of Illinois College of Medicine, Chicago, Illinois.*

# Chapter 14

# Academic Health Center Managed Health Care Plans

*by John Edward Ott, MD, FACPE,*
*and Neeraj Kanwal, MD*

## Changing Focus of Health Care

Economic pressures, and the need to provide more personal care, emphasizing health promotion/disease prevention rather than treatment of disease, have led to a change in the focus of health care delivery. Historically, a representative sample of patients could be found in most academic health center hospitals. Lengthy hospital stays, in part for the convenience of the system, provided opportunities for multiple examinations by students, complex diagnostic and treatment plans, as well as rehabilitative, chronic, and terminal care. Students could follow the natural course of the disease and learn from patients at their own pace.

Pressures to reduce hospitalizations have radically changed procedures. Patients now frequently have preadmission diagnostic evaluations followed by admission for same-day surgery and discharge, leaving little time for student workups. The natural course of the disease cannot be observed, as follow-up care is often carried out in the physician's office. Even rehabilitation, chronic, and terminal care, traditionally provided in the hospital, are now often available at ambulatory sites, long-term care facilities, and in the home. Many procedures formerly performed in the hospital, such as cataract, laser, and arthroscopic surgery, are now done on an outpatient basis.[1-10] Fewer, but sicker, patients are being admitted to the hospital, providing decreased opportunities for learning.

Most medical care is now ambulatory based, patients seen in an office setting are more representative of the "real world" of practice, and the office is a better place to teach cost-effective care; practice management; health promotion; disease prevention; patient-doctor relationships; communication skills; social, financial, and ethical aspects of practice; and the effect of chronic illness on families. This change in educational focus requires accommodations for both the patients who are available for only short periods and are less amenable to multiple detailed evaluations, and educational pedagogy. Rapid, focused evaluations are the rule, rather than the exception. Patients with undifferentiated problems must be rapidly screened to determine those who require more thorough evaluations.

As the educational focus shifts from the hospital to the office, a large number of role model physicians, not subspecialists rotating to the outpatient setting, rather than a cadre of housestaff, are required for primary care teaching. But where will they come from? Most medical schools have relatively few primary care faculty members, and they have extensive patient service obligations already. Not only are primary care physicians in short supply now, but Colwill recently pointed out that graduates entering primary care specialties have declined 37.5 percent from 1982 to 1989.[11] HMOs and other managed care plans are a potential source of primary care role models; their visibility and changing patterns of reimbursement may result in increasing numbers of primary care physicians.

## Academic Health Center Health Plans

Academic health centers (AHCs) might consider three types of arrangements with HMOs or other managed care organizations (MCOs) to generate referrals, revenues, and educational opportunities:

■ An AHC-sponsored HMO or MCO that is owned and managed by the AHC.

■ An AHC-affiliated HMO or MCO that has a contractual relationship for educational purposes but is not owned or managed by the AHC.

■ The marketing of integrated tertiary care medical services linked in part with educational opportunities for health professional students.

The most appropriate choice requires a careful analysis of the objectives of the AHC and the MCO. If the AHC is to participate in managed care, it must adapt to the rapidly changing competitive world of medical practice; managed care will not continue to accept the AHC's inefficiencies and higher costs for medical services that are readily available elsewhere. In most instances, the AHC's former trainees are now practicing in nearby suburban community hospitals, which are often more modern, more convenient, safer, and cheaper, making it more cost-effective for the MCO to contract with suburban specialists and hospitals than with the AHC unless the MCO perceives other benefits.

Before an AHC considers sponsoring its own MCO, it must clearly define its objectives, because an academically based MCO is an extremely complex source of conflict within the faculty, may compete for financial resources initially, and yet may be critical to the AHC's future. Possible objectives include:

■ Maintain or increase market share by increasing the primary care patient base; this objective is critical if the AHC depends on MCO referrals, which can be channeled elsewhere when a lower price is offered. It takes a large primary care base to provide a significant number of tertiary care referrals.

■ Improve access and referrals to the health care system by providing additional entry points through a decentralized MCO.

■ Improve patient care services by transferring appropriate inpatient and routine emergency care to more appropriate, less costly ambulatory settings.

■ Reduce the university's health care costs by providing care for university faculty, staff, and students through a university health plan that provides incentives to receive care at the AHC.

■ Bond the voluntary faculty to the open staff university hospital by involving them in the university's MCO, thereby decreasing the threat of a university-based HMO to its alumni and encouraging a long-term relationship with the medical center.

■ Contract with affiliated community hospitals to provide secondary care that will reduce hospital costs for the MCO while providing an increased number of tertiary care referrals to the AHC.

■ Use the MCO as a focal point for ambulatory teaching so that the AHC hospital can concentrate on teaching highly trained tertiary care specialists in a downsized, efficient hospital.

Many organizational issues must be considered before embarking on an AHC-sponsored HMO. The chief executive officer (CEO) of the medical center must be a "strong leader" who can foster support of key departments (ideally medicine, pediatrics, family practice, OB/GYN, dermatology, orthopedics, and ophthalmology) for the concept. The CEO should offer each department the right of first refusal to provide services, provided they are patient-oriented and cost-competitive, but not a guarantee of the business. Forcing an unwilling department to provide service results in dissatisfied patients who are treated as second-class citizens with inappropriately restricted access to care. The knowledge that the MCO can go elsewhere for services provides a strong incentive to negotiate appropriately and to compete on service. Similarly, hospital administration must contract at a financially attractive discount or lose the business to community hospitals.

The prudent CEO recognizes that the MCO needs to be an integral part of the medical center, as it will be the revenue generator for the university's evolving competitive medical organization, while the hospital moves from its traditional role as a revenue generator to a cost center.[12] The differing objectives of the HMO, hospital, and faculty practice plan are at times at odds but need to be respected. Marketplace changes occur rapidly, so the MCO must maintain flexibility and rapid decision making capability to meet the competitive challenge. Conflicts predictably arise in the attempt to balance the educational, research, and financial interests of the faculty with the service needs of the MCO.[13] The MCO's resources must be balanced carefully to benefit the medical center while maintaining a competitive premium and accommodating the innate adverse risk selection caused by patients attracted to an AHC-sponsored plan. It is better to contract at market rates and then explicitly subsidize education and community service at a fixed percentage of premium than to bury ever-increasing costs in an escalating premium.

A separate corporation, which can be controlled by the university, is required for a federally qualified HMO and is desirable to minimize interdepartmental conflict over resource allocation. If the plan is properly capitalized, the MCO should generate its own revenue through premium dollars and need not compete with other parts of the medical center for resources. If initial capitalization is inadequate, the only other sources of capital are nontaxable bonds or conversion to a for-profit corporation that can initiate a joint venture with a financial partner or make an initial public offering. The MCO is not likely to generate sufficient expansion capital from current premium dollars. One potential source of capital could be the faculty practice plan itself, which could invest in the plan in exchange for a higher payment for services or for dividends. Natural tensions between the faculty and the plan may decrease if the faculty benefits from profits of the plan as well as the provision of medical services. Board members from the faculty must be chosen carefully to ensure that they can rise above their vested interest. Universities are often uncomfortable functioning as an insurance company, even though it can purchase reinsurance to minimize that risk, and may be unduly concerned about a for-profit subsidiary's effect on its non-profit status. A rapid decision-making process that is much more time sensitive than the usual university procedures is essential to adapt to the rapidly changing competitive environment.

As a rough estimate, $10 million over the first five years will be required to obtain an insurance or HMO license, provide the necessary insurance reserves and operating capital until break-even point is reached, recruit experienced HMO executives, and develop management information, marketing, and administrative systems. It is prudent to have cash or cash equivalents equal to at least one month's total premium income to pay current operating expenses. If the university name is attached to the MCO, the university is ethically, if not legally, liable for financial losses if the plan fails. On the other hand, use of the university name is important for marketing purposes, as it implies quality as well as the backing of a stable institution.

Well-qualified, experienced MCO executives, such as the CEO; the medical director; directors of finance, marketing, operations, management information systems, and underwriting; and an actuarial consultant, need to be identified. Few of these executives have academic credentials, and even fewer will understand AHCs. These executives are in short supply and are likely to require higher income packages, including higher annual raises, bonuses, car or car allowances, and other benefits, that the university doesn't normally provide. The university community must accept advertising and marketing as appropriate functions.

The AHC needs an infrastructure that supports a suitable delivery system for caring for large numbers of patients. Primary care faculty in family practice, medicine, and/or pediatrics need to coordinate services. Teams consisting of faculty, residents, and physician assistants or nurse practitioners, who devote most of their time providing continuity of care for their patients and educating health professional students are commonly used. Subspecialty-oriented faculty seeing patients a few sessions a week are not satisfactory substitutes for primary care physicians; they generate higher costs for ancillary studies and cannot provide continuity of care.

A higher pay scale than that for similarly qualified research faculty will be required in order to meet the growing shortage of primary care physicians, as will a mechanism for recognition, promotion and tenure, or the availability of a non-tenured clinical track, which primarily rewards service and teaching. Relatively large numbers of specialty referrals for mundane services will be required in OB/GYN, dermatology, orthopedics, and ophthalmology. Some faculty seek tertiary care but have more difficulty managing large numbers of routine referrals. The health plan needs to provide routine services by using the most appropriate, cost-effective providers, such as podiatrists, optometrists, psychologists, and social workers, which may pose problems for some senior faculty members. A plan for caring for patients at suburban medical centers using faculty or contracted independent physicians is necessary to serve a broad geographical service area. Referrals from full-time faculty are easier to control than those from independent practitioners. Tertiary referrals occur most rapidly when the medical center controls the primary care patient base.

The AHC and the MCO need a management information system (MIS) with sophisticated cost accounting and management data functions, which will be useful in improving outcomes of care and reducing costs. Typical AHC MIS systems are financially driven and do not provide the management information required to administer the plan.

Faculty members have more difficulty relating to an AHC-sponsored health plan that is part of the family. Until recently, many faculty members have been isolated from external competitive pressures and the financial consequences of their own practice patterns and inefficiencies. Faculty members also have a limited understanding of the coordinating roles of primary care physicians and are offended by utilization review nurses attempting to decrease lengths of hospitalization in specialty areas where the faculty members are experts.

Faculty members may demand coverage, such as unlimited mental health or rehabilitation services, when they know that these plan benefits are expressly limited. If they are able to dictate coverage, the ability of the plan to remain competitive is severely compromised. Providing uncovered benefits jeopardizes the plan's financial condition and creates adverse risk by making premium rates less competitive. Coverage issues must be determined by market forces consistent with state and federal legal requirements. Faculty members often can accept these limitations better from an unknown insurer than from a member of the family.

Another factor affecting the premium is dysfunctional role behavior. Primary care physician faculty members may hold the gate open rather than face the displeasure of specialists who complain about unnecessary referrals while continuing to see patients on a discounted fee-for-service basis. For the system to work well, primary and other specialty physicians, the hospital, and the health plan must share the risk at all levels. Paying the specialty group a capitation payment, but allowing individual physicians to bill fee-for-service for services rendered, creates perverse incentives that result in increased premiums. All component parts must share the risks and the profits if the medical center is to survive. Unrealistic premium rates result in healthy patients leaving and sick patients remaining in the plan. A representative cross-section of patients is necessary for survival of the plan.

The long-term collegial relationships between a medical school faculty and its AHC-sponsored MCO requires careful selection of faculty, extremely good communication between the two groups, the ability of the HMO to remain somewhat distant from the faculty practice plan and hospital, and a mutual respect for the conflicting but overlapping objectives of the organizations. To date, no AHC plan has fully achieved these objectives. There is a critical need for operational independence of the various elements of the medical center. Too close a relationship compromises the MCO's ability to meet consumer's and employer's needs, because faculty are less likely to be responsive to service-oriented needs in response to complaints from the family unit. At the same time, each organization needs to recognize its interdependence with the other units.

If the AHC-sponsored MCO is held captive by the faculty or hospital, its long-term financial future and service orientation is severely compromised. In only rare instances should the CEO of the medical center be required to mediate or arbitrate disputes. The longitudinal use of an external consultant may be helpful in assisting AHC constituents to understand the inevitable conflicts and find appropriate ways to ameliorate them. One source of stress is the shift of control of both patients and finances from specialists and hospitals, the strengths of AHCs, to the health plan.

Because of the complexities of an AHC-sponsored MCO, the capitalization and managed care expertise required, and organizational concerns, an AHC-sponsored managed care program is best reserved for medical centers committed to use the managed care plan for educational purposes and for those that cannot afford to have their limited primary care patient base compromised.

The George Washington University Health Plan (GWUHP) exemplifies an academic health center-sponsored HMO. It was founded in 1972 as a wholly owned and managed subsidiary (501(C)(4) not-for-profit corporation) of The George Washington University. GWUHP is a federally qualified HMO serving the Metropolitan Washington, D.C., area. The president of the university appoints a simple majority of the board of directors and the vice president for medical affairs serves as the President of the board. One-third of the board members are consumers. The plan serves the commercial D.C. market, not just faculty and staff of the university.

The original purposes of GWUHP were to:

■ Develop a high-quality, cost-effective, prepaid health care delivery system for a heterogeneous patient population.

■ Educate health professional students.

■ Conduct clinical research studies.

The plan evolved out of a need to provide more ambulatory teaching (primarily but not exclusively primary care) experiences for health professional students. There were no economic reasons for establishing the plan. The university hospital was full, and faculty members had all the referrals they desired. The plan only needed to be economically self-sufficient and meet the school's educational needs.[14]

A single ambulatory center located near the medical center was staffed by full-time faculty members who provided both primary and other specialty medical services. Hospitalizations occurred at the university's hospital. The CEO of the medical center determined that all departments would contract with GWUHP. Only the price was negotiable, and, if the price were not appropriate, the vice president for medical affairs would establish the price (that was never necessary). The university hospital was paid on a competitive per diem basis.

The plan broke even with an enrollment of 12,500 patients in 1977 and continued to grow slowly. Competitive pressures in the early 1980s resulted in a stable, aging population of approximately 20,000 members. The plan's premium increased from the lowest to the highest in the area. At the same time, the university hospital census and number of referrals began to decline. The medical center administration recognized that GWUHP would have to increase its enrollment dramatically, operate in a niche market with an ever-increasing subsidy, or go out of business. The AHC recognized its need for additional referrals but was unable to provide the expansion capital required. Therefore, it sold an 80 percent interest in the plan to a proprietary hospital chain. The hospital chain was to provide expansion capital, additional management resources, and a new management information system. The university was to continue to use health plan facilities for educational purposes and receive a long-term service contract. Both partners made a commitment to enlarge the plan rapidly and build suburban medical centers to complement the main downtown facility.

It sounded too good to be true. It was. The joint venture was a disaster financially and administratively. The university repurchased the plan and assumed responsibility for its expansion in 1987. At that time, enrollment had increased to 26,600, but the plan was losing money at the rate of $600,000 a month. The plan, which had a positive net equity of $4,500,000 prior to the joint venture, now had a negative net equity of $4,500,000.[6]

In the past five years, GWUHP has grown from 26,600 to 54,000 members and has increased the number of medical centers from one to five. The plan has been transitioned from a group to a network model in which about 70 percent of the practice currently remains with the university. GWUHP also contracts with a relatively small number of carefully selected independent practitioners, many of whom also participate in the AHC's teaching programs, and about a dozen community hospitals. The plan is stable administratively and financially. It competes successfully in a competitive commercial marketplace while fulfilling its educational and research missions.

## Academic Health Center-Affiliated HMOs
The differing business objectives, knowledge, and experience of AHCs and MCOs, as well as the late entry of AHCs into most markets, is likely to lead more AHCs to affiliate with MCOs for education and service contracts rather than own and manage their own MCOs. In arranging such a contract, it is critical that the AHC identify a stable partner who is interested in a long-term relationship and will not cancel the contract just because a competitor offers a slightly lower price. To accomplish a long-term relationship, the differing objectives and constraints of AHCs, teaching hospitals, and managed care organizations must be recognized and balanced.

Negotiating typically revolves around issues of control; mutual and conflicting objectives; and real or perceived attitudes, stereotypes, and values. A number of authors, including Epstein, Kirz, Moore, and Ott, have discussed the advantages and obstacles to a mutually rewarding affiliation agreement.[2-6] Successful affiliation agreements recognize a mutual understanding of each other's mission and analyze the benefits each party is likely to derive from involvement in medical education.

AHCs understandably need to control the educational process in order to meet their mission and accreditation standards. There may be concerns that the managed care physicians will not be good teachers, will not understand the objectives of the rotation, and will not permit sufficient "hands on" experience to make the rotation clinically valuable to students. Consistency and timeliness of student evaluations are also a potential problem. These concerns can be alleviated by knowing the physicians and by providing orientation workshops prior to the introduction of students, as well as the establishment of a joint educational practice committee to resolve problems as they arise. Most AHCs historically have not perceived ambulatory teaching to be a priority and have not adequately budgeted for it. They now have great difficulty in reallocating educational dollars from subspecialists to generalists, especially when the generalists are not full-time faculty members.

MCOs are concerned about decreases in physician productivity; as defined by the number of patients seen per clinical session; the direct and indirect educational costs (to be described subsequently); as well as space and staffing constraints, because the managed care facilities are not usually planned with educational activities in mind.

The MCO is concerned about patients' acceptance of students' role. Patients are in more control of their participation in the ambulatory setting than they are in hospitals. MCOs must protect the consumers' right to refuse student participation. Administrators are also concerned about the number and size of the electives, the objectives of the rotation, and their costs and benefits. An agreement to share the direct expenses of the educational experience is appropriate, because all parties can benefit from the arrangement.

Each organization contributes to the affiliation agreement. The AHC expects access to large numbers of primary care patients and subspecialty referrals for tertiary care. The AHC-affiliated health plan will be perceived by the public to offer high-quality care based on current scientific knowledge. This perception is multifaceted. High-quality care is important but may lead to adverse selection when patients who are seriously ill join the managed care plan knowing they will be sent to the university hospital for their tertiary care. The AHC can also offer clinical (voluntary) faculty appointments; university hospital staff privileges (if it is an open-staff hospital); use of the library, faculty club, or other facilities; continuing medical education opportunities; credits and discounts; short-term residency exchanges; and collaborative research opportunities. Exposure of residents to the managed care plan makes it easier to recruit and retain physicians, which may be more important to the plan than a social obligation to train physicians, given the declining number of available primary care physicians. The academicians may contribute studies of clinical outcomes or cost-effectiveness of care.

The AHC will need to significantly discount its services to be competitive and to compensate for overutilization of ancillary services. It may also be able to offer malpractice insurance to the plan through a self-insurance trust at a favorable rate. The two organizations may be able to reduce redundancy of staffing and duplication of expensive equipment by joint recruitment of subspecialty faculty and joint purchases of expensive equipment, such as MRIs. The MCO also may engage in activities such as financing new practice sites, providing panels of patients for new practitioners, and offering office management consulting services or educational opportunities, which increase referrals to the university-related hospitals but do not violate safe harbors identified by the federal Medicare fraud and abuse law.

MCOs have much to offer the AHC. They can provide large numbers of patients who receive most of their care in a closed system for a given period, which is ideal for carrying out drug trials or epidemiological studies. Volunteers for most studies can be recruited without difficulty. Access to such a population may increase the likelihood of a research grant being funded. Some MCOs may have sophisticated management information systems available that collect data for business purposes that can also be useful in research and make it easier to identify patients for research protocols. The MCO can also provide a large number of primary role model physicians for the students. Students are likely to increase the physician's enjoyment of practice, lead to continuing learning, personal professional satisfaction, increased prestige for the physician, and increased recruitment and retention of physicians.

Under the right conditions, educational opportunities can be provided for students at any level of training but there are real costs involved for medical students and junior residents. The more advanced the trainees, the more likely residents' service will cover these costs, but primary care services do not generate the income that services provided in the hospital do. Realistically, it is unlikely that the AHC will be able to pay the full educational cost of teaching at the HMO, but that should not prevent satisfactory negotiation of the affiliation agreement if the managed care plan sees other benefits from the arrangement. Payment symbolizes the importance of the educational experience provided by the managed care plan and is probably not a major source of income.

The third and frequently the most difficult obstacle to overcome in negotiating an affiliation agreement is the perceived attitudes, stereotypes, and values of each organization. The AHC values the educational environment, supports research, and provides high-quality care, but commonly does not value patient care and service, while the HMO values convenient access to care and provision of cost-effective, high-quality comprehensive care that promotes health and prevention in a situation where member service and satisfaction is of great concern. Each institution's rewards reflect the institution's values, which in turn determine individual physician attitudes and behaviors.

Academicians often perceive that ambulatory patients have problems that will not interest students and HMOs as cost-cutting organizations that yield inferior care. Primary care physicians may be considered less scholarly and may generate concern about teaching ability. MCOs view AHCs as expensive, inefficient, and unconcerned about patient service or expenses. They also are concerned about loss of control and "stealing" of patients when they are referred to the AHC. Voluntary faculty are frequently discriminated against in terms of admission priorities and operating room time.

These issues, although thorny, can be alleviated by clarifying and respecting the values of each organization and the objectives of the affiliation agreement. An ongoing joint practice/educational committee to review problems and resolve them promptly when they arise is critical to a long-lasting, mutually satisfying affiliation agreement.

## Marketing of Integrated Tertiary Care Services

AHCs are increasingly marketing integrated tertiary care services at a fixed price. These services typically include all physician, ancillary, and hospital services required for a complex procedure, such as a coronary artery bypass or organ transplant. The packaged price may include transportation and a hotel room for the patient's spouse as well. AHCs are in a particularly good position to offer these services if they carry out significant numbers of these procedures and can demonstrate good clinical outcomes.

To date, the primary motivation of AHCs to package medical services has been to increase market share. It is possible, however, that AHCs could provide more favorable terms for these services in exchange for access to and participation in primary care educational experiences.

## Cost of Medical Education—Who Will Pay?

Costs of medical education emphasizing primary care and physician productivity in HMO settings have been studied using time-motion studies or time-log diaries, direct and indirect cost allocation, and marginal cost accounting techniques. Allocation of costs is complex, because it is difficult to separate clinical care, teaching, and research when they are occurring simultaneously.[15] Other factors affecting the cost of education include the numbers and training levels of the students, the frequency of the rotations of students and teacher, and the type of clinical experience (observation, "hands-on" clinical, use of a primary care teaching lab with its models, simulated or programmed patients, computerized patient management problems, or an HMO orientation seminar). Patients may also be scheduled at a more leisurely pace to permit more time for education.

Given the confounding variables and the different methodologies utilized, it is not surprising that study results vary significantly. Unfortunately, many of the published studies have an inadequate discussion of the relevant confounding variables, which makes it difficult to extrapolate the results. Subjective factors, such as patient satisfaction and the attitudes of physicians and staff, should also be considered.

Kirz *et al.* conducted a marginal cost study of the educational programs sponsored by the University of Washington at Group Health Cooperative of Puget Sound (GHPG), an AHC-affiliated HMO.[4] Subjectively, they assessed the satisfaction of physicians, nurses, and patients with the educational process. Because GHPG is a large, stable, staff model HMO with relatively fixed revenues and expenses, the researchers concentrated on assessing the opportunity costs of education. A marginal cost analysis was used to calculate physician labor, overhead, and "out-of-pocket costs." Physician labor costs were determined by counting the change in patient visits with and without students. Overhead costs per visit were calculated including nonphysician labor, space, utilities, maintenance, pharmacy, and laboratory, but do not include marketing or other administrative costs. Out-of-pocket costs were those charges actually paid by GHPG, such as stipends, books, or student parking fees. Physician labor costs in dollars were estimated using the number of direct teaching hours (not involving direct patient care) and the physician's hourly rate. A total of 201 or 10.7 FTE students in the 1982-83 academic year were evenly split between primary care and specialty care departments.

Results of the surveys indicated 98.2 percent of physicians and 92.6 percent of nurses were most satisfied with the educational arrangement. Physicians felt the students added to their enjoyment and professional education, while the nurses were less impressed. Analysis of clinic schedule logs indicated a decrease of 1.04 visits/half-day session attributable to the presence of students. The average time spent in direct teaching, which did not include personal time, lunch hours, or time before or after clinic, was 46.8 minutes per half-day. Providers perceived that the students affected the quality of care positively. Ninety percent of all patients were satisfied with trainee involvement. How many patients declined to participate in medical education activities is unclear. In total, the estimated costs of student involvement in the 1982-83 academic year was $16,900 (1983 dollars) per FTE student per year.

Stern *et al.* estimated the cost of educating 22 primary care residents in two fee-for-service hospital outpatient departments and two HMO settings, using a cost allocation method for determining direct and indirect costs as well as revenue generated from primary care clinic time.[16] All ambulatory teaching time, including that in subspecialty clinics that did not generate revenue, was included. Residents averaged five patient visits per session during the three-year residency program, compared to 8 visits per session for attendings. Residents generated roughly 77 percent of their ambulatory training costs.

Studies of physician productivity and direct and indirect cost allocation in an academic primary care department in which teaching, research, and patient care occur simultaneously and are equally important, and the marginal costs of superimposing a clinical rotation on a practice that assumes no responsibility for curriculum development or administration, have all been used to study the cost of educating junior clerks at GWUHP.

Lindenmuth examined the affect of third-year clinical clerks on physician productivity.[17] The physicians logged the number and lengths of sessions and the number of patients seen. Patient satisfaction studies were also conducted. The authors reported the number of patients seen in the student/preceptor team increased significantly from the number seen by the physician alone. However, the baseline activity of this practice assumed the presence of students and was down-scheduled accordingly; therefore, it did not represent a true potential productivity. The authors indicated the increased number of patients seen was due to seeing predominantly patients with a single, well-defined acute problem.

Pawlson *et al.* used the joint cost allocation methods developed by Carroll to determine the costs of education in the same academic department. Logs were maintained by physicians during two interspersed junior clerkships. Faculty physicians spent 22 percent of their clinical time teaching an average of 1.45 students per session per physician, or 31 minutes per one half-day session teaching students. The total cost per student was $54.20 per day or $27.10 per session in 1978 dollars.[18]

Pawlson and Watkins examined the marginal costs of instruction at the Group Health Cooperative of Puget Sound, GWUHP, and the fee-for-service offices of practicing physicians.[19] Elective clerkships in family medicine at the first-, second-, and fourth-year levels and the required third-year primary clerkship at GWUHP were studied. An incremental cost approach was used, with the assumption that patient care is the most important "product" in most practice settings. The number of patient visits before, during, and after the presence of students was used as a proxy for physician productivity.

There was no decrease in physician productivity in the first-year student family practice (FP) rotation, which was an observational experience. However, preceptors spent 0.5 hours per day longer in the clinical session when students were present. The extra time was donated by the physician out of personal time. Nurses generated a cost of 4.50/day in overtime attributed to students in 1980 dollars, which was paid by the plan. The second-year family practice clerkship decreased the number of patient visits by 8.3 per session, with a resulting daily cost of $112.00 in 1980 dollars.

The third-year primary care clerkship at GWUHP is a "hands on" experience. No increase in physician productivity occurred when students were not present, as the established productivity standards assumed the presence of students at all times. The baseline productivity at GWUHP was significantly lower than that at Group Health Cooperative. Assuming the difference in productivity between the two HMOs was due to the constant presence of students at GWUHP, a loss of 5 visits per day results in a cost of $82.00/student/day in 1980 dollars that is attributable to the third-year clerkship. One important variable between the two sites was that the physicians at GWUHP were general internists while those at Group Health Cooperative were family practitioners. An additional examining room for each student and a small conference room was necessary.

A study of private practice preceptors also was carried out; 1.2 patient visits per day were lost where students participated, at an average charge of $25.00 per 20-minute visit or $30.00 per day in 1980 dollars.

Fourth-year family practice electives at Group Health resulted in a significant loss of patient visits, at a cost of $64.01 per student per day in 1980 dollars. The preceptors felt more space was necessary. They could not maintain their full schedules and supervise senior students.

Kahn *et al.* used a work sampling technique to evaluate the direct costs of advanced pediatric and internal medicine residents who elected to work in a prepaid group practice.[20] The authors concluded that the resident physicians' productivity was comparable to that of the attending physicians and that residents' services paid for the loss in faculty productivity. This study did not take into account the need for additional facilities, nonphysician labor, overhead, or program administration costs. Neither residents nor faculty were required to see large numbers of patients, as the clinical site was underpopulated and had small patient volumes, which makes it difficult to extrapolate the results. However, a busier site should have increased productivity of both resident and attending physicians.

HMOs or other MCOs can realistically provide a controlled setting for health professional student education at any level of training. The likelihood of burnout and the negative impact on physician productivity can be minimized by having attending physicians teach intermittently, decreasing the expected number of patients to be seen according to the level of student training and increasing productivity expectations when students are not present. The experience is uniformly rewarding for teachers, students. and patients.

To be equitable, the AHC should pay at least the marginal costs of education so these costs are not passed on to patients. (Some HMOs allocate a small percentage of premium for educational and community service activities that might be used partially to subsidize these activities. Federal grants supporting primary care and family practice residencies can be used to subsidize curriculum development and longitudinal rotations in subspecialty clinics where the resident does not generate income. Research or foundation grants may also be available to support start-up costs or research products.[21]

## Summary

The focus of medical care and education is now at the ambulatory level. AHCs are well prepared to teach tertiary care in hospitalized patients but are less prepared and inappropriately budgeted to emphasize primary care, ambulatory-based teaching. Few AHCs have large numbers of primary care faculty members, and the few they do have are usually overly committed to service activities.

Joint ventures involving AHCs, HMOs, and other MCOs are a pragmatic way to involve significant numbers of primary care physicians as educational role models in "real world" practice. Depending on the specific objectives of the AHC, the institution might consider sponsoring an MCO, affiliating with a MCO, or selling packaged tertiary care services at competitive prices that include access to the MCO's facilities and to primary care physicians.

Affiliation agreements are increasing in popularity as MCOs recognize the growing shortage of primary care physicians. There are advantages and disadvantages to the arrangements, but both organizations have more to gain than lose. MCOs may be more willing to contribute financially to the educational process as they stabilize financially and understand the advantage of recruiting selected physicians whom they helped train. Negotiating issues are typically those of control, mutual and conflicting objectives, and attitude and values as perceived by the two institutions. These issues, although thorny, can be alleviated by clarifying and respecting the values of each organization and the objectives of the affiliation agreement. HMOs will probably be more willing to share in the direct costs of education in the future than they have in the past.

# References

1. Bentley, J., and others. "Education in Ambulatory Care—Financing Is One Piece of the Puzzle." *New England Journal of Medicine* 320(23):1531-4, June 8, 1989.

2. Epstein, A., and Pollock, D. "The HMO and the Academic Medical Center." *HMO Practice* 2(4):133-8, July-Aug. 1988.

3. Hoft, R., and Glaser, R. "The Problems and Benefits of Associating Academic Medical Centers with Health Maintenance Organizations." *New England Journal of Medicine* 307(27):1681-9, Dec. 30, 1982.

4. Kirz, H., and Larsen, C. "An Independent HMO's Affiliation with a University." *HMO Practice* 2(4):129-32, July-Aug. 1988.

5. Moore, G. "Health Maintenance Organizations and Medical Education: Breaking the Barriers." *Academic Medicine* 65(7):427-32, July 1990.

6. Ott, J., and Blatt, B. "The Rise and Fall of a Joint Venture: University Based HMO and a Major Medical Corporation. *HMO Practice* 2(4):147-50, July-Aug. 1988.

7. Perkoff, G. "Teaching Clinical Medicine in the Ambulatory Setting: An Idea Whose Time May Have Finally Come." *New England Journal of Medicine* 314(1):27-31, Jan. 2, 1986.

8. Swanson, A. "HMOs Have an Educational Obligation." *HMO Practice* 2(4):125-8, July-Aug. 1988.

9. Davidson, R. "Changes in the Educational Value of Inpatients at a Major Teaching Hospital: Implications For Medical Education." *Academic Medicine* 64(5):259-61, May 1989.

10. Woolliscroft, J., and Schwenk, T. "Teaching and Learning in the Ambulatory Setting." *Academic Medicine* 64(11):644-8, Nov. 1989.

11. Colwill, J. "Where Have All the Primary Care Applicants Gone?" *New England Journal of Medicine* 326(6):387-93, Feb 6, 1992.

12. Ott, J. "Competitive Medical Organizations: A View of the Future." In *Paying the Doctor—Health Policy and Physician Reimbursement.* Westport, Conn.: Auburn House, 1991, pp. 83-9.

13. Ott, J. "Administrative Medicine." *JAMA* 268(3):332-3, July 22, 1992.

14. Pawlson, L., and Kaufman, R. "HMOs and the Academic Medical Center." *Health Care Management Review* 7(2):77-80, Spring 1982.

15. Carroll, A. *Program Cost Estimating in a Teaching Hospital.* Washington, D.C.: Association of American Medical Colleges, 1969.

16. Stern, R., and others. "Graduate Education in Primary Care: An Economic Analysis." *New England Journal of Medicine* 297(12):638-43, Sept. 22, 1977.

17. Lindenmuth, N., and others. "The Effect of Third-Year Clinical Clerks on Physician Productivity in a Primary Care Practice." *Journal of Medical Education* 53(4):357-9, April 1978.

18. Pawlson, L., and others. "Medical Student Instructional Costs in a Primary Care Clerkship." *Journal of Medical Education* 54(7):551-5, July 1979.

19. Pawlson, L., and others. "The Cost of Medical Student Instruction in the Practice Setting." *Journal of Family Practice* 10(5):847-852, May 1980.

20. Kahn, L., and others. "The Cost of a Primary Care Teaching Program in a Prepaid Group Practice." *Medical Care* 16(1):61-71, Jan. 1978.

21. Ott, J. "Medical Education in a Health Maintenance Organization: The George Washington University Health Plan Experience." *HMO/PPO Trends* 5(2):6-11, June-July 1992.

*John Edward Ott, MD, is Chief Executive Officer and Neeraj Kanwal, MD, is Medical Director, The George Washington University Health Plan, Washington, D.C.*

# Chapter 15

# A Strategic Planning Model for Successful Academic Health Center Patient Care Interventions

*by Elaine King Miller, PhD, Kimball Austin Miller, MD, MSHA, Andrew E. Accardi, PhD, and Dala R. Jarolim, MD*

## Introduction

This chapter will comprehensively review the process used by academic health service institutions to determine the product or group of services they will develop and provide for their patients. The chapter will define and determine the sequential interactions of environmental opportunity analysis, strategic·intervention planning (marketing mix analysis and implementation strategy), and intervention monitoring. The chapter format will be a progression from global concepts to specifically defined steps, with examples from academic medicine.

The planning and implementation of successful health care interventions begins with an in-depth study of the needs, wants, and demands of the various consumers, organizational members, and payers. This in-depth review of service selection, organizational adaptability evaluation, and resource determination (environmental opportunity analysis and planning) is followed by a discussion of the intervention planning, financial viability determination, and marketing process used for service implementation. Finally, the chapter reviews the process for sustaining a high-quality patient care service intervention and monitoring procedures used in the modification of the health care service that are needed in this rapidly changing and turbulent health care market.

## Overview

The problem of initiating and sustaining academic health care interventions relates to the ability of the clinical organizational unit to carefully analyze potential opportunities in its external environment and to develop a strategic plan for an intervention that is consistent with the organization's other functional areas and its overarching or principal mission. The organizational unit can vary in size from a small primary care section or outpatient clinic to a substantial division or clinical department within a large academic organization. However, for efficient planning, the unit must be specifically defined with regard to purpose and relationship to other organizational units.

Extensive analysis of potential service opportunities is now considered a mandatory management function in the competitive and resource-limited health care market. It allows the institution and the organizational unit to review all segments of the internal (functional groups within the institution/organizational unit) and external (groups and coalitions not directly related to the institution/organizational unit) environment and to develop a service or group of services that fill the needs, wants, and demands of all consumers and payers of health services. Its overall value to the organization is based on its ability to identify opportunities and threats. Once implemented, the model requires scheduled, mandatory reevaluation and modification that reflect changes in environmental influences. The revolutionary rate of change in the health care environment now compels formal, semiannual reviews and constant environmental scanning to maintain a close alignment of the health care unit with all segments of the internal and the external environments in order to provide a high-quality service with perceived high value.

Traditionally, the aspects of quality in health care delivery have been defined in professional and technical terms. However, in the academic environment, new definitions of quality of care and the methods to measure it dominate the literature. These commitments to quality will be integrated throughout the organization by appearing in strategic planning and specific health care delivery models. It will become paramount for organizations to conduct ongoing, comprehensive self-assessment activities that support the principles of total quality management and continuous outcome improvement.

Effective management of health care interventions requires that the organizational unit relate to a broad and increasing number of consumers and payers, including, at a minimum, patients, parents or guardians, physicians, nurses, federal and state regulators, employers, certifying and accrediting organizations, alternative health care delivery systems, public and private third-party payers, business health coalitions, and integrated hospital systems. All these participants of the external environment are integral to the development of a successful intervention or service and will determine if a program has targeted the appropriate group of consumers, has the potential to be reimbursed for its services, and has the ability to survive and prosper.

The traditional business strategic intervention plan for designing the marketing mix for a service is appropriate for use in the health care industry. This planning model includes:

- Definition of the specific product, service, or group of services that the subunit of the organization will provide to the consumers.

- Determination of the place and distribution channels for the service.

- Performance of a pricing analysis to determine the relationship between price and demand, the existence of substitutes, and the cost of complements that could affect demand for the proposed service.

- Determination of the appropriate mix of advertising and promotion that will inform target market segments or consumers of the existence of providers who will perform the service that consumers are ready, willing, and able to demand.

This intervention is based on a knowledge of the organization's physical structure and professional resources and capabilities. Institutional strengths and weaknesses and professional adaptability influence the choice of opportunities and resultant strategies that have a high probability for success. Each organizational unit must extensively analyze its structure, areas of effectiveness and strength, and known vulnerabilities and weaknesses to be able to develop a successful intervention. In an academic health care intervention, the physical environment and format of health care delivery is crucial to the primary, secondary, and tertiary care patient; therefore, organizational resources and staff member creativity, empowerment, and adaptability must be at a high level to obtain a successful intervention and take advantage of the broad possibilities of innovation and change.

Although the strategic intervention planning component of the model is based on the four major instruments of marketing mix analysis (products/service, place, price, and promotion), academic health care interventions must also conform to the values and mission of the organization's internal environment or culture and the norms and mores of society. Many governmental and not-for-profit health care organizations perceive that health care services are a basic right of the individual and therefore are not items that should be looked upon as subjects for analysis, planning, and marketing strategies. However, in an increasingly competitive and resource-limited environment, the use of a strategic planning model is appropriate because it allows for efficient use of scarce institutional and governmental resources to address the needs and wants of all consumers. Current resource reality demands an understanding that wants are unlimited but means are not. Consumers and payers must determine the best allocation of their limited financial resources and therefore must be informed of their options and the cost/benefits of their service choices. Only informed consumer and payer groups will force the health service provider to constantly evaluate and modify its intervention programs. If this model is implemented, it will result in efficient provision of health care services, an organizational orientation toward consumer satisfaction, and favorable institutional asset turnover, cash flow, and net profit.

## Environmental Opportunity Analysis— Organizational Response to the Environment

There are numerous points from which to view the health care organization's response to its environment. The traditional business organizational behavior model views the environment from two perspectives: its rate of change and its degree of homogeneity. By rate of change, we refer to the relative degree of stability and flexibility in the environment. The degree of homogeneity refers to the complexity of the environment. It is a simple environment if it has few unchanging elements and virtually no segmentation, or it is substantially complex when there is a large number of rapidly changing elements and the environment is vastly segmented. These two factors combine to determine the level of uncertainty faced by an organizational unit.

Uncertainty can be a powerful force that drives any number of decisions made by the organization. The least amount of environmental uncertainty will be faced by health care organizations with stable and fairly simple environments. However, it is important to realize that no current environment is devoid of uncertainty. The academic environment bears its unique type of uncertainty: residents, students, and faculty all at different levels of knowledge, patients of all socioeconomic backgrounds with various levels of compliance and understanding, changing federal and state regulations, evolving requirements of the Joint Commission on Accreditation of Healthcare Organizations, and complicated medical patient problems referred to the "medical experts."

Organizations with volatile but simple environments tend to face moderate uncertainty. Organizations with stable but complex environments similarly experience moderate uncertainty. As might be suspected, organizations with very volatile and unstable segmented environments are complex and will, therefore, face an extremely high degree of uncertainty. The clinician manager must understand the service unit's organizational behavior and response to uncertainty when planning a new service intervention to promote its strengths and minimize its weaknesses as it moves away from the secure and familiar.

A more pragmatic measure of the organization's strengths and weaknesses is determined by its response to competitive forces. A specific method by which to assess the organization's ability to interact with its environment is its actions and new service interventions while being threatened by specific competitive forces. The traditional five competitive forces are:

- Threat of new entrants.

- Jockeying among contestants.

- Threat of substitute products.

- Power of buyers.

- Power of suppliers.

Each organization or unit can analyze and assess its internal environment quite effectively through measurement of its response to environmental uncertainty and its ability to respond to traditional competitive forces. The academic health care unit uses these measures as the initial foundation to determine its ability to consider a service change or develop a new clinical service. An organization should only start the next step of environmental opportunity analysis if it can accept some environmental uncertainty and be willing to interact with competitive forces. All members must understand and accept that some people will lose power, influence, or status; others will have to learn new skills and behavior patterns, work in new environments, and associate with new and different people. The academic health care unit must create win-win situations where team members can grow and be successful in response to change.

## Environmental Opportunity Analysis— Segment Evaluation and Planning Framework

In academic health care, an environmental opportunity analysis, followed by specific program planning should be a group process where service providers evaluate all segments of their internal and external environment in a stepwise manner to develop steps that result in a plan or strategy for service implementation. To survive, succeed, and sustain institutional programs, the organizational unit must:

- Understand its target markets or groups of consumers and payers.

- Understand its interaction with other portions of the organization.

- Identify and utilize organizational unit synergy and alignment with the organizational global mission.

■ Obtain and develop the needed resources (human, financial, physical, informational) to produce the service.

■ Accept organizational unit change and the concepts of continuous quality improvement.

■ Determine if the institution or organizational unit has the resources to promote a high-quality product or group of services efficiently and effectively.

■ Develop a cost-effective implementation strategic plan to distribute these services to the appropriate consumers in a timely and professional manner.

■ Develop a management information system that can integrate financial and clinical data while continuously monitoring resource use.

■ Review the effect of future health care trends on the proposed new service.

An opportunity analysis needs to delineate the synergy expected to result from organizational decisions related to changing markets, resource development, and areas where the organizational unit has specific or unique expertise. The first step in achieving this organizational objective depends on the identification of a range of academic health service opportunities that are congruent with the mission and goals of the institution. The mission or principal goal of an organization is molded by three elements. The foundation, or first element, is the history of the organization's aims, policies and accomplishments, while the second element is the current dominant preferences of senior management. The final element is the institution's resources and current areas of special competence. All these elements fuse into the determination of a principal mission. The global mission statement of the institution usually will not only set the organizational tone but also limitations on service provision and target populations or service groups. An intervention plan that does not consider organizational goals and the program objectives of other functional areas of the institution will be inefficient, possibly redundant or in conflict, and often short-lived. It must be supported up and down the organizational hierarchy and have its health care activities designed to strengthen the solidarity of and organizational commitment to the overarching mission.

Once the organizational environmental evaluation is completed, analysis of other external environments can proceed. This analysis attempts to determine the range of specific health services that fulfills the needs and wants of the patient, the learner, the teacher, the researcher, and the third-party payer. Health care institutions or agencies usually produce services and not products. Services are described using the variables of time, energy, and skill. When deciding on the array of services to be provided, the provider must recognize that services are intangible, inseparable from the provider, and perishable. The output of the organizational unit cannot be stored and is totally dependent on the provider and consumer because the production and consumption of the service occurs simultaneously. If the appropriate mix of services is chosen and the other instruments of intervention planning are accurately determined, these services will be accepted in the marketplace by providers and consumers with minimal promotion.

Effective methods of determining consumer interest include direct surveys, focus group studies, and complaints/suggestions correspondence. For example, a selected sample of patients who complete a survey or participate in focus group discussions can be questioned about their interest in specific health care topics and health related problems, in addition to demographic and socioeconomic determinants. Within each potential service area, adult consumers are asked to rate their interest on an ordinal scale relative to their views of the service (positive versus negative) and the potency of their views (strong versus weak). From the data generated by this instrument, the planner can select potentially promising services for further evaluation to align the health care organizational unit with environmental opportunities.

The next stage of the opportunity analysis determination is selection of which services should be targeted toward each potential specific segment of the population. Target marketing analysis allows for three general methods of segmentation. Product/market concentration consists of the organizational unit's focusing on a specific service in only one segment of the patient population.

An example of opportunity analysis-segment determination of this concentration model would be study of the feasibility of implementation of a mammography screening service and the selection of mammography equipment at a university internal medicine ambulatory care center. Analysis of information from consumers, providers, referral sources, and competitors would show:

■ Physician offices and multispecialty groups are potentially major mammography providers and referral sources for women in all age groups.

■ The demand for these screening services has been shown to increase directly with household income.

■ Household income has also been known to affect consumers' selection of the facility from which to seek health services.

■ Women in higher income households tend to use private physician offices more frequently than do women from lower income households, who tend to use university ambulatory care facilities.

■ All consumers, but especially lower income consumers, prefer services conveniently located, with high value and low cost.

Therefore, after analyzing the demographic and socioeconomic composition of the patient population cared for at a university internal medicine ambulatory care center and at potential competitors in mammography services, a low-cost, spartan, but convenient screening service would be subjected to intervention planning and financial viability analysis.

Product specialization consists of focusing on a specific service, but designing the program for the provision of this service to several segments of the academic health care population. An example of this would be development of a physical rehabilitation clinic that could also address the exercise and fitness boom. More physical therapy is being offered in ambulatory centers, and it is expected that this trend will continue as providers expand their delivery base to meet the needs of an increasingly fitness-minded society.The multifaceted service would be designed to provide specific physical therapy to inpatient and outpatient orthopedic and neurologic patients and have the flexibility to offer sports medicine, general physical fitness education, adult cardiac rehabilitation, and exercise programs for children, adolescents and adults.

The third type of segmentation is a market specialization model that consists of determining a specific population segment and providing all or most available services to that population. An academic medicine example for this demographic segmentation model would be a women's health care center with services ranging from general medicine/gynecologic care through weight loss/sports medicine and programs for every aspect of what differentiates the female throughout her life cycle. The woman's differing emotional needs, responses to stress, and responses to drugs and alcohol could be considered when providing services through the university women's health center.

Targeted consumers must be analyzed for buyer behavior characteristics if the academic health provider is to have a successful and sustainable service. Traditionally, analysis has focused on the behavior characteristics of the patient or legal guardian. However, with the rapid development of alternative health care systems, business-health coalitions, and managed health care forms of medical insurance, the wants and goals of commercial, not-for-profit, and governmental payers must be thoroughly considered.

Specific competitor behavior also should be evaluated at this stage of analysis. Competitors' market share, current profitability, and cost of service provision must be documented, and an assessment of current patient satisfaction should be obtained. If possible, trend analysis should be completed to determine the responsiveness of these competitor health care organizations to prior demographic, economic, regulatory, reimbursement, and social value changes that affected this consumer segment. This detailed selection of segments of the population and specific services (as opposed to attempting to provide a complete array of services to all portions of the population) will help the organizational unit survive by providing it with potential flexibility to modify its portfolio of services and targeted market segments while providing profitable service interventions.

The second part of the environmental opportunity analysis is initially oriented toward groups outside the provider unit to determine the current feasibility and need for development of the service. Once this foundation is completed, the next step is to look again within the organizational unit to identify its specific strengths and weaknesses and to determine if the professionals within the unit have the ability and resources to develop, maintain, and distribute the specific health care services. This analysis must be objectively completed using a self-study model and perhaps using an outside independent consultant. Current physical environment, financial, and professional time allocations must be determined, and their priority compared to the new service must be acknowledged. This is especially important if the new service is a vertically integrated activity rather than a diversification type of venture in order to promote smooth interactions and transitions for optimal service provision and cost efficiency.

At this stage of the planning process, it is useful to evaluate the product/market opportunity matrix. This matrix forces the organizational unit to look at different opportunities and the resources needed to achieve each option. When implemented, new services can be promoted in new (total innovation) or current (product innovation) market segments. In general, the implementation of a new service to an old or current market requires fewer resources and has a lower level of uncertainty than the initiation of a new service into a new market. Therefore, in the planning stage, the total resources necessary for each choice should be calculated and the impact on the total resource allocation of the organizational unit should be evaluated. An academic medicine example of product innovation might be the initiation of outpatient counseling services for the current patients of a general internal medicine practice, while total innovation would be its development for residents of an adult day care center located near the general internal medicine practice or the acquisition and management of a nursing home practice.

If resources would be reallocated because of integration or diversification strategies, leaders must determine if this reallocation would have detrimental effects on other current programs, if the professional and support staff are in agreement with the new priorities of the service-providing unit, and the effect of change on the provider staff. It is usually appropriate to develop a collective ownership of the new priorities through the provision of a mechanism for staff input and feedback. Further, if it is determined that new staff would be needed to implement the service program, there should be a clear understanding of the responsibilities of these new team members and their direct and indirect interactions with the current staff. The time and effort expended during this phase will yield substantial benefits through producing a unified and goal-oriented team, inclusive of administration and clinical staff, focused on the established priorities. With this collective focus and use of participative management, the group is able to progress to the final step of the environmental opportunity analysis.

The last step in the opportunity analysis and planning process forces the health care administration professional to evaluate future primary care health care trends within and outside the organization. As a result of the prior stages, there should be organizational agreement on the specific service that will be provided, determination of the targeted health care consumer segments that will be receptive to the defined services, and identification of the resource allocations that will be required to develop, maintain, and distribute the service. Before developing the strategic intervention plan, there must be an evaluation of predicted influences (social, economic, demographic, technologic, governmental, and competitive) that would change the marketplace characteristics or needs and wants of consumers, providers, and health care payers.

Examples of current changing health care variables that could affect academic medicine would include changing reimbursement policies, changing and expanding health education programs, increasing use of home diagnostics, changing government regulations, competitive sealed bidding per patient for a given diagnosis, dwindling philanthropic sources, changing grant funding emphasis, increased managed health care protocols, increased emphasis on outcome measurements, extension of fixed payment systems, changing allopathic and osteopathic specialty physician supply, fewer medical students opting for primary care residencies, decreasing autonomy expectations of academic health professionals, influx of international medical graduates, and the effect of long-term health promotion and disease prevention programs.

Therefore, potential environmental changes must be considered in this planning stage and a determination made to see if they would affect the adaptability and survivability of the proposed service and the global objectives (academic goals, survival, patient care growth, high-quality service, profit or increased reserves, consumer goodwill, and management flexibility) of the institution. The proposed service must allow for management flexibility to realign with a change in the environment. The organization cannot react to the changes, threats, and opportunities with denial or opposition. Only through modification and adaptation can it react successfully to environmental challenges and flourish.

In summary, there are multiple dynamic forces that interact in a complex manner to affect the outcome of the academic health care environmental opportunity analysis. In addition to internal and external environmental forces and resources, provider flexibility and ability to face uncertainty must be taken into consideration and incorporated into the planning analysis. The overall objective of the environmental opportunity analysis program is to define the targeted population or group of consumer needs, wants, and interests and to develop a general service delivery compatibility model that determines if the provision of this mix of services results in optimal benefit to and satisfaction of consumers, providers, and the organization.

## Strategic Intervention Plan

The final result of the environmental opportunity analysis stage provides the information foundation needed to design the specific intervention plan for the implementation of a new academic health care service. The transformation in type of information has been from global generalized ideas to specific finite determinations regarding new services and target markets or consumer segments. The first stage of the strategic intervention plan is called marketing mix intervention analysis, the function of which is to obtain an objective decision process to implement a service activity on a schedule, within budget forecasts, and with ongoing evaluation protocols. The traditional four "Ps" of the analysis mix are product or service, place, price, and promotion. However, for health care in general, because the output of the organizational unit is usually a service, a fifth "P" (people) must be added to the intervention analysis.

Because the character and quality of academic health services are inseparable from the providers that deliver the services, the fifth "P" must be the first area of the analysis. Health care services are an interactive activity that depends on the personal relationship between the health care provider and the patient. The service is produced and consumed concurrently and is highly variable, depending on the provider of the service and integral support staff team members. Therefore, at this stage of the analysis and planning, the organizational unit must specifically determine which members of the health care team will interact and deliver the services to the target population. Team selection must include all professional and full- and part-time support staff members who will interact with any consumer segment, be it patient, parent, referral source, or payer. Administration must develop selection practices to screen for aptitudes, skills, attitudes, and personality traits and select team members able to move away from the secure and familiar and change existing programmed behavior. Personnel budget determinations must be planned, and staff compatibility must be evaluated. Objective behavioral and performance goals and rewards should be determined in writing at the outset to promote, both financially and psychologically, desirable behaviors while eliminating nonconforming behaviors during probationary periods with outplacement counseling. The team philosophy must reflect a customer-oriented emphasis and culture.

Each member of the health care service team must view the provision of the service as a team effort and must coordinate his or her activity with other members. This service focus can be achieved if team members are chosen so that there is congruence of the organizational unit goals and the individual member aspirations and goals. This alignment philosophy must be evident within all levels of the clinical, administrative, and support staff, with the desired behaviors becoming a way of life and expressions of personal as well as organizational preference. Once such alignment is achieved, it is helpful if a team member is assigned responsibility for facilitating continued consistency of beliefs, values, vantage points, and goals during the implementation and service delivery process.

The products of clinical academic health care organizational units usually include health status assessment, acute medical illness evaluation and treatment, chronic illness management, behavioral assessment and treatment, preventive health services, and health education. These products, which benefit several parties in the interaction, are often intangible and usually do not result in the physical transfer of an object from one party to the other. Services cannot be packaged, counted, and stored; however, the product is measurable through the physiological and psychological benefit obtained by the patient and his or her family and the education of the medical student or resident.

Although there is a benefit to the consumer, the demand for the service can be negative or positive in nature. A negative demand for a service is a situation where the consumer dislikes the service and will avoid it, even though it will result in a personal benefit. Examples of negative demand services in health care are immunizations, dental work, and chemical usage evaluations. A positive demand for a service occurs when there is an active interest in the product or service. Medical examples such as ulcer treatment and acute respiratory illness management typify services provided to patients that are both desired and beneficial. Therefore, in the intervention planning analysis, there must be quantitative measurement and documentation of the magnitude of demand and the benefits derived from each service or product for each consumer segment.

The specific resources necessary to provide the individual service must also be determined. This cost will depend on the volume of services provided, so a determination must be made for different volumes of service and the cost per service must be calculated. Because volume will depend on the service's position in the product life cycle, its current position should be located on the curve and a prediction of the rate of change should be estimated. Product life cycle theory views the service or product as having an expected growth and decline cycle.

There are four stages of product life: introduction, growth, maturity, and decline. During the introduction stage, volume typically is low and cost per unit is high. This is a time when the staff must work out technical and information system problems, because the next stage is growth. During the growth stage, there is a rapid increase in the volume of clinical services provided and a drop in the cost per unit as the organizational unit benefits from economies of scale. There is a drop in the rate of growth as the service unit goes into the maturity stage. During the long maturity stage, there is minimal to no growth in the volume of service provided by the organizational unit. Volume is at its maximum, and the average cost and marginal cost per unit (additional cost to produce the next unit of service) is at a minimum. The service that is being provided is well developed and vulnerable to challenge from newer clinical interventions. When this occurs, the service is in the decline or final stage of the product life cycle.

With the average and marginal cost projections calculated for the clinical service within the growth and maturity stages, the organizational unit can address the issue of service price. In determining the price of the clinical service, three areas of analysis must be addressed: pricing objectives, pricing strategy, and market segment differential pricing. The area of price objective uses the basic microeconomic concepts of supply and demand and elasticity of demand to determine price while taking into consideration the organizational objectives of ideal consumer usage and acceptable return on investment. Surplus or profit maximization is achieved when pricing is set to enhance the difference between price and costs. Using the microeconomic supply and demand equation, this would be at the volume with minimal cost, with the price set at a level such that demand is equal to or greater than supply. This determination depends on the elastic nature of supply and demand. In an ideally elastic situation, there is a proportional decline in demand with an increase in price. However, in health care, inelastic demand sometimes allows an increase in price without a proportional decline in volume, resulting in greater profit or surplus maximization. This inelastic nature of some health care services exists because of consumers' positive view toward good health and aversion to death and disability, plus the lack of patient options with regard to providers of services in specific situations. For example, in elective primary care health visits, the consumer would have greater elasticity or control in the determination or acceptance of a price, in contrast to the situation where they must use health care specialists because of an accident or an acute illness.

Once the cost per unit of service (the breakeven price) and the maximum price are determined, the organizational unit must look at other factors that will affect the determination of the final charge to achieve the organizational unit objective. In price strategy determination, there are two approaches--price differentiation and quality differentiation. In price differentiation, the organizational unit attempts to become the price leader in the market segment and prices the clinical service such that its product is known for having the lowest unit price. The price is set so there will be a rapid increase in volume to achieve the optimal cost per unit volume. Then there can be a redetermination of price, depending on demand. Using the quality differentiation approach, a "community rate" pricing strategy is used. The price is determined by using the usual and customary charges of the community, and the organizational unit does not attempt to maintain a formal relationship between price and cost in its attempt to obtain its objective or profit goal. This method stabilizes the price competition in the community and does not give any health care institution a competitive price advantage in the market. Therefore, the organizational unit must use consumer-perceived quality differentiation, while maintaining the community stable price to have an advantage over competitors. Provider quality and the physical environment are promoted and consumer-oriented conveniences are implemented in this pricing strategy. The health care service unit promotes an image of up-to-date technology and unhurried, caring, personal attention, while filling the consumer demand for cost effectiveness and convenience. Although pricing strategy primarily looks at price and quality differentiation as the only determinants of price setting, both factors must be constantly compared to cost per unit of service to maintain the organization's financial viability.

Both price and quality differentiation are available in the open fee-for-service marketplace. However, with the increase of managed and government-sponsored health care, their effects are blunted. Market differential pricing occurs when there is acceptance of external environmental controllers of pricing in specific market segments. Because health care service charges are regulated in many areas by rate setting agencies and determined through negotiation with large commercial insurance companies and alternative health care delivery systems, the imposed or negotiated price for the particular service can be unrelated to cost. Therefore, the price charged can differ for each market segment and payer. In summary, pricing is determined by reviewing organizational profit objectives and analyzing cost, demand, and competition, with the final price influenced by mandated regulation and/or negotiation with third-party payers and alternative health care delivery systems. However, the final price must allow for an acceptable return on capital investment and cover all direct and indirect operating costs.

The third "P" (place) is especially important to the time-limited adult patient. Therefore, in strategic intervention planning, there must be an evaluation of how the services will be made available to the targeted health care market segments. This evaluation activity has two components--physical plan location and structure and time management. Determination of patient traffic and activity patterns will indicate opportunities for location of the organizational service unit if new construction is contemplated. The range of options considered should include a building adjacent to current campus facilities, a single tenant office building near the campus, a large community employer-based facility, a shopping mall leased area in the local community, a multispecialty office suite in the community health plaza, and a mixed-use office building. Other factors that must be considered include current and predicted competition in the area, location of major educational and recreational facilities, projected demographic composition of the area, location of major employers that provide insurance benefits, and proximity to inpatient and laboratory facilities.

The structure must be distinctive, but it must also conform to the norms, mores, values, and needs of patients. Convenience to transportation must be considered, as well as vehicle parking and structural lighting for security. For example, the availability of public transportation could be important to one group, while the availability of secure parking is mandatory to another. The physical structure and interior decoration must reflect the norms and values of the target market to promote acceptance of the service. If a new physical structure is not being considered, location or relocation of the unit within the institution must be evaluated considering access, confidentiality, and potential signage.

The internal physical environment of the service-providing unit should be coordinated by a professional interior designer cognizant of current design trends and preferences of the patient population. Office furnishings, written educational material, and video entertainment in the waiting room should be appropriate for the age and the educational level of the selected patient population. The dimensions of the service unit should also be appropriate for the predicted volume during the early growth phase and easily expandable for expected utilization during the mature phase. The internal design should promote confidentiality and efficient patient flow and allow for adequate waiting areas, exam room space, inventory/storage areas, and conversational/counseling offices. Overall, the environment should promote a professional atmosphere that reinforces the feeling of high-quality care, service value, and comfort. The design should promote a positive mood for faculty, staff, learners, patients, and their families.

It is also important to emphasize that the physical environment encourages staff members and care providers to convey a service orientation in interactions with patients. The development of a service orientation involves the deliberate design of an organizational culture and facility that sanctions a service orientation and understands its relationship to the survival, growth, and maturity of the organizational unit and the future employment of all members of the health care team. The planning of the physical environment should involve staff members in service delivery at all levels, drawing on the human creativity of the organization to achieve a collective goal.

Time management aspects of the intervention planning process relate to hours and days of operation, office waiting time duration, and appointment waiting time length. Academic health care service providers must be sensitive to barriers to service that can exist if hours of operation are limited and waiting time is perceived to be of long duration. Services should be provided in a timely manner and should be available during times of easy access for all members of the patient's family. The schedules of providers must allow for enough face-to-face time to build a doctor-patient relationship and promote consumer satisfaction. Constant monitoring of consumer feedback is essential. Every effort must be made to promote access and convenience to patient populations with diverse life-styles and time schedules.

The last "P" in the marketing mix intervention analysis is promotion. This aspect of intervention has undergone significant changes over the past two decades, from using professional referral networks, word-of-mouth communication, and general public topic awareness methods to sophisticated multimedia advertising campaigns integrated with rebate and reward programs. All new service units use open house events, basic informational advertising in appropriate medical and health professional publications and newsletters, and visibility at professional educational meetings. Further, it is customary to provide basic descriptive material to various health professional and community groups and to discuss proposed new service interventions with key health agencies in the community and the region.

Any activity beyond basic advertising depends on the norms and values of the organization and of the professional societies in the region. What might be considered appropriate in one geographical area could be trivial or overzealous in another location. Examples of successful patient advertising range from simple radio and newspaper informational messages to coordinated efforts with other hospitals, county health departments, athletic sports stores, fitness centers, and the like. These activities can be coordinated with current news topics or can be related to a local or regional health-promotion activity. Typical examples would include writing a health column in a community newspaper or having faculty interviewed monthly on the local television health education program. Further, it is now customary for health professionals to be guest speakers on nightly news television, at regional or community functions, at in-service programs for allied health professionals, and at community government meetings.

The final result of the sequential environmental opportunity analysis and marketing mix intervention analysis is a specifically defined implementation strategy (second component of the strategic intervention plan) for the proposed service in the targeted market segments. All constituencies of the internal and external environments have been analyzed, and relevant needs, wants, and desires have been addressed and satisfied. Participative management systems and techniques for adapting to environmental changes have been implemented to promote long-term survival and growth. The organizational unit is now ready to deliver the service more effectively and efficiently than its competitors. The final test for a strategic intervention lies in the implementation strategy's ability to survive and succeed in the targeted market while achieving organizational pricing objectives.

## Sustaining and Monitoring Interventions

Strategic planning must play a critical role in the management of any organization. All institutions must develop short- and long-term strategies to respond to the rapidly changing health environment. Every health care organizational unit has strengths and weaknesses and is presented with opportunities and threats. Although much of the institutional energy and resources are expended on environmental and market analyses and intervention implementation stages, for survival and growth, the organization must allocate effort and resources to the monitoring of the intervention and its interaction with the internal and external environments. The intervention monitoring program must have universally known procedures to resolve internal problems, whether personal, interpersonal, intragroup, intergroup, or organizational in an open climate in which differences are confronted, clarified, and resolved. The monitoring system must give direct feedback on all aspects of the intervention and all members of the staff while evaluating the financial viability of the intervention and promoting continuous quality improvement.

A major aspect of monitoring is market share analysis. This determination allows for a comparison of the organizational unit and its competitors regarding relative market share. Comparison of market shares must be evaluated as a function of the current situation and evolving trends since implementation of the new service. Three factors (volume, cost per unit, and market share) allow the organization to evaluate its ongoing performance and deviations from model projections. They form a clear objective database for higher levels of the organization to compare different organizational units, allow prioritization of total institutional resource allocations and form the foundation for projections that will be used during the next evaluation period.

This process can be demonstrated through consideration of implementing a mammography screening service in a government rate setting environment. Success requires an adequate volume of patients. If 12 women on average are examined each day, approximately 3,000 mammograms per year will be performed. Assuming that about 40 percent of eligible women will avail themselves of the service, a population of 7,500 women over the age of 35 would be required to provide the necessary number of patients. If the target population has only 15,000 such patients, the organizational unit must have a 50 percent market share.

The second factor of monitoring relates to the overall profitability of the intervention and the auxiliary services that are generated by the existence of the intervention service. The profit or loss determination must be undertaken for each target segment at projected and actual volumes and must be analyzed in comparison to prior periods. Institutional standards of minimum profitability are usually used as a basis for comparison, and pruning of unprofitable population segments (if possible) can allow for survival of selected target segments or groups of segments. Although a service might be provided efficiently to a large segment of the population, overall profitability must be achievable for survival. An analysis of the financial feasibility of the intervention will not only enable prediction of financial success, but also assist in readjusting the price to the proper level. Once projected expenses have been determined and the number of anticipated procedures have been established, a charge for the service can be calculated to ensure profitability and determine the survivability of the service.

An academic medicine example would be to reevaluate an unprofitable satellite clinic to determine more appropriate service delivery in terms of hours of operation, staffing, and administration. Consideration of integrated units and associated profit centers should be taken into account when analyzing the profitability of the satellite clinic. Furthermore, a determination of service compatibility is important for internal environmental harmony and for promoting the overarching or principal mission of the organization. The health care service, if vertically integrated, must facilitate efficient transfer of patients and resources while having a positive effect on contiguous units. Because of possible unit myopia, this determination must be done objectively by internal or external professionals who are knowledgeable of the total mission and goals of the organization and all of its units. Determination of compatibility with the external environment must include measuring of the satisfaction of all consumers' needs and wants. This evaluation tends to improve the level of service and promotes professional gratification and workplace contentment.

Finally, the maintenance stage of intervention monitoring is crucial to the continued health of the organization. With the current revolution in health care, obsolescence of policies and strategies is inevitable. The adaptive organization is constantly repositioning itself to promote efficiency, value, quality, and performance while actively exploring new services that meet current and potential patient, family, and payer needs.

## Conclusions

Analysis, planning, implementation, and sustaining of successful academic health care interventions require an in-depth study of the needs, wants, and demands of internal and external environments relevant to the organizational unit. Emphasis must be placed on analytical procedures of environmental opportunity analysis, marketing mix intervention analysis, and implementation planning. The organizational unit, whether a small primary care clinic or a department of a large organization, must identify opportunities and risks in terms of consumers, the organization, its competitors, and society. Members of the service unit must develop a joint ownership of the potential opportunity and promote a coordinated dual authority (health care providers and administrators) to implement the changes needed to achieve the desired goal. Once the unit determines that there is a consumer need and want that it can effectively and competitively satisfy, it must evaluate this potential opportunity regarding the specific issues of people, place, price, product, and promotion. All organizational units that pursue consumer needs and interests find that innovations designed to promote consumer satisfaction create opportunities for growth, image enhancement, outcome improvement, and alignment of provider and consumer desires. However, any implementation plan, no matter how well conceived or effectively implemented, must adapt to the responses of the target population and fulfill organizational profitability requirements. Further, to survive and prosper, the unit must constantly reevaluate the health care service and its congruence with the current and future desires of the target population and the evolving organizational mission.

## Bibliography

Albrecht, K., and Zemke, R. *Service America!* Homewood, Ill.: Dow Jones-Irwin, 1985.

Augustine, N. *Augustine's Laws.* New York, N.Y.: Penguin, 1987.

Bolman, L., and Deal, T. *Modern Approaches to Understanding and Managing Organizations.* San Francisco, Calif,: Jossey-Bass, 1986.

Boss, R. *Organizational Development in Health Care*. Reading, Mass.: Addison-Wesley, 1989.

Bradford, D., and Cohen, A. *Managing for Excellence*. New York, N.Y.: John Wiley & Sons, 1984.

Califano, J. *America's Health Care Revolution*. New York, N.Y.: Random House, 1986.

Coile, R. *The New Medicine*. Rockville, Md.: Aspen, 1990.

Dolan, R. *Strategic Marketing Management*. Boston, Mass.: Harvard Business School Publications, 1991.

Drucker, P. *Innovation and Entrepreneurship*. New York, N.Y.: Harper & Row, 1985.

Dyer, W. *Team Building: Issues and Alternatives*. Reading, Mass.: Addison-Wesley, 1977.

Griffin, R. *Management*. New York, N.Y.: Houghton-Mifflin, 1990.

Ishikawa, K. *What is Total Quality Control? The Japanese Way*. Englewood Cliffs, N.J.: Prentice-Hall, 1985.

Joint Commission on Accreditation of Healthcare Organizations. *Principles of Organization and Management Effectiveness*. Oakbrook Terrace, Ill.: The Commission, 1989.

Kolb, D., and others. *The Organizational Behavior Reader*. Englewood Cliffs, N.J.: Prentice-Hall, 1991.

Kotler, P., and Clarke, R. *Marketing for Health Care Organizations*, Englewood Cliffs, N.J.: Prentice-Hall, 1987.

Kotter, J. *Organizational Dynamics*. Reading, Mass.: Addison-Wesley, 1978.

Mintzberg, H. *The Nature of Managerial Work*. Englewood Cliffs, N.J.: Prentice Hall, 1980.

Ouchi, W. *The M-Form Society*. Reading, Mass.: Addison Wesley, 1984.

Peters, T., and Waterman, R. *In Search of Excellence*. New York, N.Y.: Harper-Row, 1982.

Peters, T., and Austin, N. *A Passion for Excellence*. New York, N.Y.: Random House, 1985.

Seay, J., and Vladeck, B. *In Sickness and in Health: The Mission of Voluntary Health Care Institutions*. New York, N.Y.: McGraw-Hill, 1988.

Suver, J., and Neuman, B. *Management Accounting for HealthCare Organizations*. Chicago, Ill.: Pluribus Press, 1986.

Wolinsky, F., and Marder, W. *The Organization of Medical Practice and the Practice of Medicine*. Ann Arbor, Mich.: Health Administration Press, 1986.

*Elaine King Miller, PhD, is Associate Professor, Department of Management, College of Business, Colorado State University, Fort Collins, Colorado; Kimball Austin Miller, MD, MSHA, is Associate Professor, Departments of Internal Medicine and Pediatrics, Section of Health Care Design, College of Medicine-Tulsa, University of Oklahoma, Tulsa, and Adjunct Professor, School of Health Administration and Policy, College of Business, Arizona State University, Tempe; Andrew E. Accardi, PhD, is Administrator, Clinics Administration, University of Oklahoma Health Sciences Center, Tulsa; and Dala R. Jarolim, MD, is Chief of Medical Services, Veterans Administration Medical Center, Tulsa, Oklahoma.*

# Chapter 16

# Academic Health Centers and the Future of Health Care

*by Ralph E. Horky, MHS,*
*and J. Richard Gaintner, MD, FACPE*

**M**assachusetts politician Thomas P. ("Tip") O'Neill made the observation that "all politics is local." In at least one sense, it is fair to say that health care is also local. The call for a "National Health System" notwithstanding, the essential health care relationships are varied, intimate, and one-on-one in nature. Over time and through repeated contact, a level of mutual understanding and confidence is established between a health professional and a patient. This fundamental continuity is necessary for high-quality outcomes. What is now called "case management" has always been a formula for high-quality care.

Even as health services delivery becomes more "corporatized" and more "merchandized," case management principles are still an integral part of the picture. Even large multispecialty group practices and million-subscriber health maintenance organizations have institutionalized an economic model of the case manager as a means of controlling costs in their broad and diverse delivery systems. The "primary care gatekeeper" is, at its basis, a modularized version of the family " doc." Because this personal consultative relationship has been persistent and valued, it should be a part of any effort aimed at improving health care services.

Similarly, a "rational" and convenient system of hospitals is a necessary component of any solution. That system should manage care at all institutional levels—from maintenance to critical intervention—and should ensure an available bed for any patient in need of it. Doctors need a principal practice site for patients whose conditions are serious or who otherwise need close and continuous observation. The aging population may portend even greater need for such institutional services. While the number or types of beds needed may be debatable, the concept of institutional care remains valuable and relevant. In fact, as "easy cases" are relocated to more economical surroundings, residual inpatients are sicker and more costly to treat on a per patient basis. Unfortunately, ensuring access to doctors and beds is simply not enough.

During the past two decades, a massive economic restructuring of the American health care system has occurred. Most of the activity has been in tangential spurts of regulatory action aimed largely at the institutions of medicine or at its practitioners but seldom at both. Because there are relatively fewer institutions than doctors, regulatory actions targeted at hospitals have been relatively more successful than those directed at physicians. This is not to say that doctors have gotten off scott free, but they have been less affected by "outsiders getting into their business." (In this undistinguished category, doctors may be catching up rapidly.) In the past 20 years, health care costs have risen in every measurable category.

Throughout this period, change in the professional culture of medicine has lagged behind the tremendous change experienced by the corporate culture of health institutions. Put another way, the institutions of medicine, the workplaces, have migrated down from very different paths from their most important workers, the physicians. Hospitals and doctors have always had somewhat different agendas. Today, they seem barely able to comprehend each other's problems fully.

It is thought that academic health centers (AHCs), and especially the medical schools with which they are closely tied, have an important cultural influence on medicine. This influence is purportedly based on the persuasive power of scientific truths and scholastic values. These truths and values have, at least traditionally, transcended economics. The degree to which this cultural influence can or should be parlayed into real operational leadership is the subject for the body of this chapter.

By way of introduction, it is the authors' belief and thesis that the requirement to continually reconcile the needs of institutions with the cultural expectations of the medical profession has become a core problem in health policy, institutional management, and health system design. This "problem of communication" lies in the critical path of the health care industry's ability to self-regulate, to establish strategic direction, and to distribute social responsibility. We predict that the quality of the future of health care will be derivative of the quality of the adaptation of the physician culture to more structured workplaces and work methods.

Because this change may cut to the very source of physicians' professional esteem, understanding the physician culture is a necessary first step to creating an environment for constructive change. Understanding the variety and motivations of institutions is equally essential. Each of these variables will be examined singly and in relation to the others. Finally, because America's academic health centers are at least the unofficial stewards of medical culture, it is necessary for them to accept a leadership role.

## The Physician Culture

Attributes of the ideal doctor have been well described by great physicians, such as William Osler. Even in the 1990s, it is worth rereading such insightful philosophical pieces as his essay "Aequanimitas."[1] The doctor comes to the patient interaction without a cluttered mind. He or she listens! With careful closure against the contaminating distractions of previous encounters and other events of the day, the patient is observed and offered individual attention, discretion, and counsel and the benefit of accumulated scientific knowledge.

Such consulting relationships are the essence of case management. They require a doctor's mindset and a practice environment that respects the style and nature of that intimate interaction. Privacy is needed. Communication links to colleagues and libraries are important, but the intimidating presence of blinking computers in the examination room is hardly conducive to personalized care. The commercial environment of meeting halls, gray corridors, and laboratory vestibules piled with strange and distracting equipment is neither optimal nor welcomed.

These principles are reemerging strongly today under new rubrics. What were formerly "good patients" have become "health care consumers." Practicing consumerism, these consumers do not wish to be viewed as objects, but rather as the owner/operators of their bodies. They want to participate in their own care as actively involved adults, not as inert scientific subjects. The concerns of consumers start, rather than end, with the technical competence of the doctor. For better or worse, consumers feel they have the right to assume competency and that they are entitled to personal service.

A second effect of "consumerism" has been to raise the popular awareness of rising health care costs. The trend toward requiring well-insured and articulate patients to expend a few dollars "out of pocket" has made it apparent that a massive superstructure of expense is being stepped down to the point of clinical service. Little else could explain such prices. Consumers want the full value of that expense: high quality, effectiveness, and a reasonable price.

Today, media stories of medical triumphs are likely to be paired with editorial sidebars on poor access, poor service, and high costs. Thus, consumer attitudes toward doctors are moving slightly out of synchronization with the physician self-image. Many doctors, especially in academic circles, do not relish the image of service professionals engaged for a fee. They have been socialized in a self-image transcending this basic level of professionalism. They have earned their position in the medical "club" and feel that, as the credit card advertisement proclaims, "membership should have its privileges."

Physicians, especially those practicing at AHCs, prefer the image of physician scientist. Biomedical scientists spar with problems having submolecular roots and international branches. Biomedical research is among the nation's few endeavors that are still regarded as having global interest, relevance, and commercial potential. In an era in which the public's image of the profession is wavering, this more heroic self-image may be defensively projected to the patients of even pure clinicians.

Since the library at Alexandria, scholars and students have known the benefits of the accumulation of knowledge and collegial interaction. Excellent science requires an elite, literal scientific community with a supporting scientific culture. The culture for inquiry tolerates uncertainty and cluttered detail. It is heuristic but carefully controlled to avoid negative consequence to patients and society. A free flow of similar but not distinct ideas is encouraged, as are generalization and speculation.

Medical research is, in fact, a tense, full-time occupation where scientific territories can be fiercely defended. To compete in the world arena, grants need be nationally competitive. Big businesses stake public and private ventures with huge investments. The growth of commercial interests and the need for "marketable" products as outcomes increases the proprietary atmosphere. The line between the academic researcher and the entrepreneur is beginning to blur as surely as is the line between the physician and the service professional as research technology transfers into commercial application.

Revolutionary advances in communication technology have not superseded the benefit of physical adjacencies for collaborating scientific disciplines. Ordinary telephone lines provide conduits for millions of observations to be transported compactly from city to hamlet. But personal direct conversation over coffee still generates the context in which science flourishes. The vast capital required to equip ultramodern laboratories and to secure and maintain biologically pristine atmospheres also argues for centralization (if not outright isolation) of the research function.

Optimum investigative environments are different from the optimum patient environment. Scientists are well supported in technologically intense downtown workplaces; conversely, active clinicians may desire more friendly, accessible environments among the patients they serve. Little place remains for general logic in most scientific settings at the senior investigators' level. The clinical world is bimodal. Generalists and specialists are equally needed, but it is the generalist who sees the most cases and the specialist who is popularly regarded as being the senior position.

Even though the environmental and personal/interactive requirements of the scientist and the physician contrast, tradition, educational paradigms, and societal expectations sustain a cultural stereotype of all practicing doctors' being facile in science and of all physician scientists' being able to draw insight directly from the bedside. Since Abraham Flexner, this complex self-image has been socialized into doctors on a wide scale through an arduous educational process that is both enuring ritual and pedagogy. Given the contrast in professional demands of the two disciplines, the frequency with which truly productive physician scientists emerge is remarkable.

Whether by personal inclination or discipline, most physicians, both primary care consultants and physician scientists, seem to covet this complex image. Both the art and the science of medicine are characteristics of their profession and requisites for their job. Medicine is distinguished as surely by the mindset of its professionals as by the challenges of human diseases.

This complexity of character, which is especially strong in physicians at AHCs, would seem to be an ideal mindset for medical case management. Situations requiring the synthesis of scientific detail and immediate observation are common in the patient care theater. Decisive physician leadership is essential. Confusion is inexcusable and can be devastating, especially at times when such decisions relate to life and death. Patients want their doctors to mix compassion and science to achieve the cure and sometimes want them to be a little larger then life. As important, it is a role model reinforced by other health care professionals who calibrate their authority against physicians' singular status.

As well defined as the physician leadership role is in the culture of medicine and in case management, it is poorly defined in the institutional bureaucracies of health care. With a few notable exceptions, the huge administrative support and logistics systems that surround patient care are usually managed for, or just as likely around, doctors. Professional administrators who are not usually physicians manage institutions. These administrators traditionally have limited direct interaction with either doctors or active patient care theaters.

This distinct separation between management of the systems that support production and the assembly process—doctors' domain of case management—is especially evident in hospitals. Having doctors so clearly dominant in one ultimately vital aspect of management and yet so remote in others produces an estrangement between doctors and their workplaces. The psychological distance between doctors and the systems of management and resource control in their principle institutions is vastly different from work relations of most other professions. The lack of linkage is a fundamental organizational characteristic that limits the ability of most large institutions to achieve any sustained strategic drive in the business sense.

In the effort to buffer the individual physician from management detail, a vital linkage and sense of commonality with the organization is lost. Not only can this be confusing and frustrating to physicians, but also it may deprive them of the opportunity to learn basic skills and concepts related to organizational behavior. Many of these concepts are so familiar that it is assumed by others that doctors fully understand them but defiantly or arrogantly refuse to incorporate them in practice.

This unusual separation may reserve physician time and energy for the demands of bench research, education, or building an ambulatory practice; however, it comes at the substantial expense of a fundamental management opportunity lost. At the practical level, no one except the physician has the "real time" opportunity to reconcile the use of resources with the demands of patients and their medical and surgical problems—to case manage—and it is the "within the case" cost, the actual cost of diagnosis and treatment, that must be understood and managed if real savings are to be achieved in the health care arena. The practical result of this cultural division is that internal "political" influence, rather then managerial leverage, unites hospitals with their means of production.

## The Character of the Institutional Base

For many decades, clinicians and physician-scientists had relatively few choices of workplace in which to base their professional practices. Those inclined toward science remained closely linked with medical schools and teaching hospitals. Those whose predominant interests were clinical left the confines of academic health centers and established themselves in communities on the staffs of general hospitals. Community physicians maintained an association with the science of medicine through former classmates and mentors, professional associations, and journals. Collegial interaction with the AHC was reflected in the referrals of complicated patients from former students to professors. This provided critical streams of revenue for the teachers and eventually medical schools.

Within the more traditional career paths, town vs. gown has blossomed into a fully diversified array of choices that are blurring the historic destination of physicians. Medical schools are, more than ever, developing primary clinical practice revenue as a means of financially supporting their scholarly missions. Accommodations with individual faculty are becoming more flexible. These alternative arrangements mix levels of academic and clinical involvement and include practice options of relative independence or in professional groups with administrative support. Social and quality of life options also differ widely. Meanwhile, community medicine is becoming much more sophisticated and "scientific." A highly technical atmosphere is attractive to the best products of America's medical schools. It is also an attractive image to patients.

Other new "alternative" delivery vehicles, which seemingly pop up daily, are not based in this culturally blended tradition. The new organizations are not identified with a single hospital nor are they based in a local perspective of community need. Many of these new care systems are capitalized business ventures competing for patients on the basis of illness type or in "niche markets." These alternative structures in health organization often have far less regard for the interdependency of the cultural needs of the profession of medicine and the structure of the workplace. They are more typical businesses, owing no strong sense of allegiance to academic attributes of the professions or to the local commonwealth. Their contributions to the economics of health care delivery have become substantial. Their contributions to the cultural wealth of medical science are marginal.

The consequences of the growth and diversification in these workplace alternatives are particularly hard on research. In the AHC, research is significantly subsidized by institutional "in kind" support, which is almost exclusively provided by the academic clinical economy and its institutions. The large general teaching hospital may be especially at peril if the economic balance shifts decidedly toward the entrepreneurial sector, because its research and teaching missions rely so extensively on the continued fiscal strength of a very narrow environment. These institutions are particularly vulnerable in regional competition!

AHCs are medicine's cosmopolitans. Component institutions may be grounded in the community, region, or state, but the AHC itself is only coincidentally an extension of those causes. With the balance of an ideal physician, AHCs respond to the art, the science, and the profession of medicine rather than geography or government. Their contribution is national and global. They are, like other great social institutions, the proper objects of support and philanthropy.

The service products of AHCs and their principal teaching hospital affiliates are profoundly different from the service products of other components of the health care system. The "flagship" academic health center teaching hospitals (AHCTHs) are health care's most completely unified organizations—crucibles of the health sciences where patient care, education, and research are blended. Elements of education, patient care, and research (and their associated costs) are amalgamated in each service product. These elements are usually inseparable and indistinguishable to patients at the point of service.

The underlying cost structure of academic medicine is complicated. The "academic medical economy" is a subset within the larger sphere of health care. Its economics support medical education, research, and advanced medical science as interdependent elements. Still, the academic medical economy is collectively dependent on and vulnerable to a general medical economy that is volatile. The terms of change for academic medicine are being dictated by the long-range economic functions of a delivery system that extends well beyond the direct influence and control of academic medicine.

Academic health centers have been the culturally richest, most prestigious, and most technologically complex of medicine's workplaces. AHCs are really multi-institutions, with a medical school and one or more teaching hospitals joined by other schools and colleges, programs in biological and technical science, graduate studies programs, and technical training programs. Some AHCs include research institutes and foundations. In short, AHCs have no definitive organizational form. They are medical "city-states," with interdependent institutions bound by common purposes and having their own social tempo, values, and mores.

More and more, traditional singular general teaching hospitals are adopting greater numbers of network affiliates in distributed locations. This trend is both a reaction to clinical competition and a practical response to training concerns. The times may dictate that the large general teaching hospital has become too expensive, too remote from everyday practice, and too complicated a "partner" to be an exclusive, or nearly an exclusive, teaching site for training in the practical aspects of early detection and management of routine care. This is not criticism. These great institutions have an irreplaceable role in the culture of academic medicine. But is it really reasonable to expect an AHC teaching hospital to ever again be "all things to all people?"

Primary care, especially preventive medicine programs, are invariably treated as "sidelines" in most tertiary hospitals. Low-intensity services are a real response to real community need but not core business. Physician education programs, as Barondess and White[2,3] have so eloquently discussed, must address both public need and science. But these vital services may be misplaced on the organizational platform of tertiary hospitals with physical plants geared to critical intervention. Consequently, they are also a questionable choice as the best, most appropriate teaching venue for these services.

From an educational perspective, "networks" of diversified teaching sites may satisfy the need for training experiences, but such sophisticated networks need to operate with high levels of formal management science. This, in itself, will exact a cultural price from academic medicine. Integration of the necessary managerial logic is a new requirement. It must sift into the already crowded and demanding curriculum for physicians in training. Physicians in practice must begin to at least understand the dynamics of organizations and management!

As businesses, AHC teaching hospitals are not clearly distinguished from their clinical "competition." With some exception for state university systems, AHCTHs leverage their human and capital assets as do other hospitals. The dynamics of general hospital management are effected surprisingly little by association with a medical school. If the medical staff is an "open" or a "mixed model," even formal and informal relationships with doctors may exist in patterns familiar to other hospitals.

Community hospitals for many decades have existed at the opposite end of the institutional spectrum from the AHCTH. Especially since the Hill-Burton legislation in the 1940s, community hospitals have been bedrock local institutions in America. The social investment in the local hospital has been so profound that it is frequently identified with the general quality of life in a community. Trustees and senior executives are typically much more involved with friends, neighbors, churches, and other local charitable agencies than with the vagaries of advanced science. Staunchly independent physicians with dominating clinical interest and strong patient loyalties populate community hospital medical staffs.

Communication regarding the referral or transfer of patients between institutions offers insufficient cultural ground to establish continuous dialogue between the physicians of community hospitals and those of AHCs. Neglect of community hospitals by the academic community has been legendary. Strong local social commitments, combined with physical and cultural distance from the medical school's "state of the art," may have had the consequence of allowing the occasional community hospital to clinically drift unnoticed beyond the means of its finances, physical plant, and intellectual and technical resources. For many years, the contrast between AHCs and local community hospitals served as a natural delineator between them. It also minimized the overlap in their societal functions and the competitive friction between them.

The notion of a large, publicly accessible health care "system" containing all types of institutions has had its strongest advocate in government regulation. In an attempt to control hospital growth and stem the costly diffusion of capital, many state governments required "demonstration of need" documents from hospitals seeking to add new technology. In theory, these documents rationalized resource use by limiting access to new technology to physicians with proven competence. In application, they caused populations to be geographically partitioned into regional health care subsystems that were mathematically delineated areas, not real communities.

This process fueled institutional competition. Community hospitals competed among themselves and with AHCTHs to become regionally designated centers for trauma, burn, imaging, open-heart surgery, lithotripsy, angioscopy, and other procedures. The theoretical "system" was illusory for doctors who continued to have their own catchment areas and referral relationships. It had relatively little impact for highly scientific and competent AHCs. They were only minimally affected by the demonstration of need documents. In slightly paradoxical fashion, they continued to exist outside systems they ostensibly personified.

Be it academic parochialism or institutional arrogance, this detachment from the system has parlayed into a deep health delivery dilemma. Teaching centers have been intent on training young doctors in the culture of scientists of the type appropriate for the AHCTH, despite a community need for generalists. Many community hospitals have therefore needed to reach to foreign markets to staff their general services. The problem that a community hospital has had attracting qualified physicians may not be viewed by academic leadership as a problem of the system, but rather may be mistakenly seen as a consequence of flaws in the management or character of the specific community hospital. High-quality hospitals, they might argue, could attract quality graduates! This is not always the case.

An abundance of young physicians with high levels of specialization and the coincidental fact that physician reimbursement schedules heavily favored procedure-oriented practices have aided the growth of high-technology "regional hospitals" outside the sphere of academic influence. Competition for AHCTHs has grown, while community hospitals have atrophied. Medical schools no longer easily entice young graduates to pursue general career tracks. Those disciplines are poorly compensated and are associated with the less prestigious hospitals. They are outside the reasonable cultural expectations of new doctors with huge student loans to repay.

Compact and reasonably affordable technology and a steadily increasing supply of community-based, board-certified specialists are bellows fanning the restructuring fires of the health industry. The growth of regional centers has proliferated the scientific aura of medicine, but it is unaccompanied by academic restraint, involvement, or overhead. Large regional patient population bases have replaced the neighborhood quality of community institutions. Mobile, sophisticated consumers convenience shop. They are not influenced by established town loyalties and are intolerant of the inefficiencies of academic settings. An important source of clinical funding has been removed from the academic economy. An ideal workplace has been created for well-trained, technically competent physicians with little regard for pomp and circumstance.

In supporting residency rotations or even maintaining freestanding residency programs, hospitals achieve a direct economic benefit. Residents still provide economical clinical coverage. The presence of residents affords the best hospital the intangible benefit of "academic patina." But the service products of most hospitals, even those with sizable residencies, are by comparison to those of AHCTHs, quite simple. They do not carry large economic burdens of medical education, nor do they have major research investments. They merely support (through technology purchases) the industries that in turn directly support research and technology development in the academic centers.

## The AHC Role in the Emerging System
After more then 100 years as the focal points of the American health care system, academic health centers are challenged to find a new place in a changing order of health science and health service. To compete with other regional care sources on a per case basis, many AHC teaching hospitals may need to reorient their work

load toward more focused clinical interests or more homogeneous patient case loads. This would allow selected services to be delivered with greater efficiency and high service quality. But the external forces of change are pressing hard to accelerate the integration of academic medicine into the nation's overall social and health service network, forcing them to become ever more general and reliant on clinical volume and revenue while capable and economical community hospital capacity is wasted. Perhaps this will ultimately result in a substantial decentralization of AHCs as network organizations.

AHCs and their most closely associated AHCTHs have moved beyond being models of exemplary applied science and sources of professorial support and have become major participants in regional and national medical economies. Their professorial and entrepreneurial roles conflict. The exercise of market power by academic institutions results in competitive reactions that ripple through the entire health care system. A new management science that is cognizant of the fundamental nature of medicine (and can be embraced by physicians) is needed to secure the academic medical culture as the delivery system continues to reorder.

Thus, in hospitals' limited role, their value is mitigated by the practices of the professionals who work there. The gap between institutional management and the medical staff is large in academic centers. It is perhaps even larger in nonacademic institutions where there are no substantial group practices or medical school faculties to provide a means to communicate with physicians as organized units. Community and regional hospitals are well steeped in the mildly extortive business practices of staff physicians who will admit their "patients elsewhere unless...." Reducing the managerial gap between hospitals and doctors is an essential first step in cost management.

Physicians can no longer treat increases in societal health care costs as being totally outside their control. Cost is not a simple function of patient demand. In that theory, the demand for personal health services would be insatiable. An appetite, to paraphrase Shakespeare, grows more intense as it is fed! Physicians are the captains that must manage case costs as well as interventional effectiveness. To have no such manager at the elemental level is a fundamental flaw.

The social need for scientific medicine that is humanely delivered is ever strong. The fact that the new order of health services is not evolving out of the culture of medicine but rather from the economics of health delivery is not a reason to disinvest in the provision of academic services. It is an opportunity to design new accommodations between the medical culture and business practice.

The responsibility for managing scientific research and medical education has been retained to a remarkable degree by practicing members of the profession of medicine. This is a unique professional attribute that is well integrated into the culture of medicine. The influence of physicians is needed to continue the societal recognition of the social benefit of academic service products.

Realignment of the institutions of health care has altered demand patterns by rerouting patients needing routine service away from community doctors and community hospitals and "upward" to clinically sophisticated workplaces and "outward" to noninstitutional care organizations. In the process, regionalized care has lost some personal qualities that are not likely to be regained. The supply of health services is artificially skewed, as affordable and accessible institutional (community hospital) capacity is wasted.

Medical school clinical practices must integrate into regional care provision. To remain educationally vital, training venues must be as varied as the opportunities for workplaces that future doctors may expect. How these practices relate to the community is critical. The competitive advantage of the academic patina is already diluted. The influence of academic medicine and the professional culture may still be preserved and even enhanced. Recognition of the value added by intensive education and research, not possession of a singular franchise with a medical school, is key to the survival of major teaching hospitals.

Physician managers can and should play key roles in these new organizational structures. The patient must be foremost as the fruits of science are delivered. The future of health care for the public is to be found in the art and science of both medicine and management. Ideally, academic health centers can remain as "beacon lights for the future and not museums of the past."[4]

## References

1.  Osler, W. *Aequanimitas: with Other Addresses to Medical Students, Nurses, and Practitioners of Medicine*. (3rd Edition) Philadelphia, Pa.: P. Blakiston, 1932.

2.  Barondess, J. "The Academic Health Center and the Public Agenda: Whose Three-legged Stool?" *Annals of Internal Medicine* 115(12):962-7, Dec. 15, 1991.

3.  White, K., and Connelly, J. "The Medical Schools's Mission and the Population's Health." *Annals of Internal Medicine* 115(12):968-72, Dec. 15, 1991.

4.  Evans, L., consultant to the Connecticut Regional Medical Program. Personal communication, 1970.

*Ralph E. Horky, MHS, is Senior Vice President for Planning, and J. Richard Gaintner, MD, FACPE, is President and Chief Executive Officer, Deaconess Hospital, Boston, Massachusetts.*

# Index